LOSE

Dr Miriam Stoppard, well-known writer and broad-caster, had been a failed dieter all her life until finally, at the age of fifty-two, she developed a diet based on sound medical know-how that helped her lose weight rapidly and then *keep it off*. LOSE 7 LBS IN 7 DAYS is the result.

She lives in London and Buckinghamshire with her husband, the playwright Tom Stoppard, and her two sons and two stepsons.

Lose 7 Lbs in 7 Days

and be Slim and Healthy for the Rest of Your Life

Miriam Stoppard

HEADLINE

First published in 1991
by HEADLINE BOOK PUBLISHING PLC

10 9 8 7 6 5 4 3 2 1

ISBN 0 7472 3565 1

Typeset in 10/12½ pt Mallard
by Colset Private Limited, Singapore

Printed and bound by
Collins Manufacturing, Glasgow

HEADLINE BOOK PUBLISHING PLC
Headline House
79 Great Titchfield Street
London W1P 7FN

For Gudrun

Contents

Foreword

The plethora of diets on the market attests to the fact that few work. As an eternal sceptic I do not make any promises that mine will succeed for everyone, but it does have certain things to recommend it. It is scientifically based. It is medically sound. It is nutritionally correct. In fact, a pregnant woman could go on to my eating plan secure in the knowledge that she would be getting all the nourishment she needs for herself and her baby. Most important, my diet stops you putting the weight back on because it introduces you to a new form of eating that is so attractive you do not want to stop. Unlike other restrictive diets, on this one you *have* to eat six times a day – which keeps you satisfied, checks your appetite and pre-empts binges.

This diet also concentrates on those foods which we all love and which most other diets exclude – the carbohydrates. If you want to have a meal that is pure carbohydrate, you can and should – it makes good dieting sense – and there are suggestions in the book about such meals. The beauty of it is that it's easy in both the short term and the long term. Using this book, you can be trim for the rest of your life.

Lose 7 Lbs in 7 Days

Confessions of a Failed Dieter

I have a vested interest in a healthy eating plan because I have been a fatty and a failed dieter all my life. At the age of fifty-three I finally seem to have cracked it – for the first time I feel free from the need to be slim. And I want to share my secret with you.

If you are overweight, you are unhealthy. So one of your goals is to be not only a trimmer you but a healthier you. I am not promising that you will live longer, but it is fairly safe to say that you will enjoy the life you have more if you are fit and trim.

As a doctor I believe that any eating plan must emphasise the long term, and, with the acquisition of new eating habits, make it easy to keep the weight off. We have to start paying attention to how we eat, how often we eat, the ritual of eating; we have to acquire a new personal psychology of eating – not an easy job when so many bad habits have to be unlearned.

Basically, my eating plan is divided into two parts: the initial strict seven pounds (pages 26–87); and the plan for the rest of your life (see pages 89–156).

Preparation is a key factor, for good preparation will help to ensure your success. The step-by-step guidelines on how to optimise your chances of success by choosing your start time carefully, signing the contract and doing all your shopping for the week will ease you into the eating plan.

The eating plan is not irksome, meals are not boring and tasteless. Great care has gone into making them delicious and attractive as well as quick and easy to prepare. To boost your morale, and as a reward for getting through the day, there is a treat for every day. Give yourself a well-deserved pat on the back, not with food, but with something else that spoils you. In addition to a treat, each day is rounded off with a tip of the day, a simple exercise of the day and a relaxation exercise.

If you stick to the eating plan, weight loss is unlikely to be less than seven pounds – it could be more. Bear in mind that if you cheat on the odd occasion it is not the end of the world.

Please do not jack the whole thing in as you have in the past. We now know that the body does not work on a twenty-four clock as far as eating is concerned, but on a much longer one, probably nearer a week. Which gives you lots of opportunity to make up for any misdemeanours.

Come on, you can do it. The key is to change the way you think. This time you will be successful – it has rarely been made easier. More importantly, it has rarely made as much sense.

Contract

I have Decided to Start on a New Eating Plan

I will decide when I am going to start and mark it in my diary.

I will make my decision public and tell my family, friends and people I work with. I will try to get their support.

I will follow the seven-day eating plan precisely, without cheating, and I will lose seven pounds in weight.

I shall seek help from . . . .
[insert name of partner or friend] who will encourage me at all times to stick to the eating plan, and whom I can call on for support.

I shall weigh myself on [date] and not reweigh myself until the seven days are over.

At the end of seven days I will get into my jeans/dress/swimsuit.

I will undertake all of these actions:

Signed . . . .   Signed . . . . . [SPONSOR]

Witnessed . . . .   Witnessed . . . .

Date . . . .   Date . . . .

You, Your Food and Diets

There has long been a great deal of confusion about the best way to lose weight and keep it off. Here are a few facts that should help to clarify the situation.

If you eat more than you need you will put on weight. The energy you need to run all the everyday processes that go on in your body is determined by the rate at which your body is 'ticking over' at rest. This is called the basal metabolic rate. It is difficult for experts to measure your metabolic rate exactly as it is a complex business. They have to know how much oxygen you inhale and how much carbon dioxide you exhale as the energy sources are burnt in your body. Plenty of energy is used, even at rest, as your heart beats, your diaphragm contracts and relaxes, your digestive system breaks down food and pushes it along, and millions of other macro and micro events take place. Quite a lot of energy is lost or deliberately burnt off as heat.

The average figures for the basal metabolic rate

of a man or woman depend on their height, weight and body composition. Body composition is especially significant and also widely misunderstood, but, put simply, it means lean muscle versus fat.

Say a lean 65 kilogram man requires about 1,500 kilocalories a day just for his basal metabolism (in other words before doing any kind of activity). Of that, the tissue mass of muscle, brain, liver, kidneys and heart will account for over four-fifths of the energy used. Since fat is not an active organ, it requires very little energy to be maintained. Now a fat 65 kilogram man would, in fact, have a smaller body mass of active organs, the difference being the extra fat. In practice most of the deficit is muscle. With less muscle and more fat, he might only require some 1,250 kilocalories a day for his basal metabolism.

And so, when you are overweight, the problem is not as simple as you may at first think. Not only do you have excess fat over your ideal weight but you probably also have fat instead of muscle accounting for some proportion of what you have discounted as your ideal weight.

Never mind, the point is this: the more muscle you lose as a percentage of your body weight, the less energy you need. But there is an answer. If you combine dieting with exercise, you will not only build up your muscle mass and tone up muscles that are out of condition, you will also raise your metabolic rate and so burn up more energy whatever else you do. Furthermore, by exercising, whether it's brisk walking, bricklaying, morris dancing or marathon running, you will burn up energy over and above your basal metabolic requirements, which means that, once your weight is satisfactory, you will be able to consume more calories as food and still stay at your ideal weight. None of this is new information but it's surprising how easily it can be forgotten when reading the hype on some of the more unlikely diet regimens.

Stop Dieting, Start Eating

As you can now understand, the amount of energy you burn daily, apart from any specific activities you undertake, is variable and you can make a positive impact on it. You can also do the opposite. The popularity of microdiets in the last few years (diets of only some 350 kilocalories a day) has prompted concern about loss of lean muscle mass rather than fat loss. But the most striking argument against them is their effect on the basal metabolism. The body put on a starvation diet thinks it really is starving and takes appropriate action. This action is akin to hibernation, although not quite as drastic. The body simply slows down and burns less energy. That is why a small woman who is heavily overweight can consume a few hundred calories a day and *still* put on weight whereas another small, heavily overweight woman eating more calories a day may actually lose weight.

My diet avoids this trap. You eat a sensible amount each day of lots of different foods – that is, small amounts of fat, salt, sugar, red meat and processed foods and large amounts of fresh fruit and vegetables, beans, pulses and wholegrain rice and oats. What's more, by eating your daily food in six meal instalments you burn off more calories than if you ate the same food as three meals.

Getting Started

Even if you are a failed dieter all your life, this time you are going to succeed. I've made it as easy as possible for you to follow my eating plan by supplying a shopping list, menus and recipes for all seven days. Each day I tell you a little more about how to use healthy foods to your advantage. I also suggest muscle-toning and relaxation exercises to get you into better shape and, because you deserve it, each day there will be a treat. Finally, I have lots of tips on how to overcome cravings and stop bingeing and even on how to overcome your doubts about completing the week or, if the worst happens, the urge to cheat.

Now, the first thing to do is take a good look at yourself the next time you're undressing. If there are bulges in the wrong places, tell yourself that soon they'll be a memory because once you've regained control you won't let yourself slip back to that situation.

Next, weigh yourself on the scales. I don't like weight watching once I've started slimming because some days I lose weight and others days I don't, which can be demoralising. The truth is, your body weight fluctuates anyway and so it's better to look at your weight from week to week rather than day by day. Far better, find a pair of old jeans or some other favourite piece of clothing that's getting a bit tight. Hang them up in a prominent place so that, each time you weaken, you can see them hanging there waiting for you to wear them.

You should know your height, but if you don't, measure that as well. Now check yourself against the standardised height/weight table (below). For each height there is an 'acceptable weight' range which is designed to cover the normal variation in body shape. Nowadays, tables are unisex with the range covering weights for small frames to large frames. If you are a woman, your ideal weight should be nearer the lower figure and if you are a man, depending on your build, the figure may be nearer the upper end of the scale. Overweight is taken as above acceptable weights and obesity as starting at 20 per cent above the upper end of the acceptable range.

Incidently, as a species we don't vary as much as some of us would like to think. There is no such thing as having 'heavy bones' and the only people who have light bones are probably suffering from osteoporosis, literally porous bones, a condition that can often be avoided if your normal diet contains enough calcium and, especially for women over the age of thirty-five, if you make sure you do a reasonable amount of weight-bearing exercise like walking, running, riding, cycling – even just standing.

Acceptable Weight Range

Height		Small Frame		Large Frame	
Metres	Feet, inches	Kg	Stones	Kg	Stones
1.45	4'9"	42	6 st 6 lbs	53	8 st 3 lbs
1.48	4'10"	42	6 st 6 lbs	54	8 st 5 lbs
1.50	4'11"	43	6 st 8 lbs	55	8 st 7 lbs
1.52	5'0"	44	6 st 9 lbs	57	8 st 10 lbs
1.54	5'1"	44	6 st 9 lbs	58	9 st 1 lb
1.56	5'1"	45	7 st 1 lb	58	9 st 1 lb
1.58	5'2"	51	8 st	64	10 st 1 lb
1.60	5'3"	52	8 st 2 lbs	65	10 st 2 lbs
1.62	5'4"	53	8 st 3 lbs	66	10 st 4 lbs
1.64	5'5"	54	8 st 5 lbs	67	10 st 5 lbs
1.66	5'5"	55	8 st 7 lbs	69	10 st 9 lbs
1.68	5'6"	56	8 st 8 lbs	71	11 st 2 lbs
1.70	5'7"	58	9 st 1 lb	73	11 st 5 lbs
1.72	5'8"	59	9 st 3 lbs	74	11 st 7 lbs
1.74	5'9"	60	9 st 4 lbs	75	11 st 8 lbs
1.76	5'9"	62	9 st 8 lbs	77	12 st 1 lb
1.78	5'10"	64	10 st 1 lb	79	12 st 4 lbs
1.80	5'11"	65	10 st 2 lbs	80	12 st 6 lbs
1.82	6'0"	66	10 st 4 lbs	82	12 st 9 lbs
1.84	6'0"	67	10 st 5 lbs	84	13 st 2 lbs
1.86	6'1"	69	10 st 9 lbs	86	13 st 5 lbs
1.88	6'2"	71	11 st 2 lbs	88	13 st 8 lbs
1.90	6'3"	73	11 st 5 lbs	90	14 st 2 lbs
1.92	6'4"	75	11 st 8 lbs	93	14 st 6 lbs

Taken from *Diet, Nutrition & Health* (BMA, 1986)

If you find you are overweight (and you probably know that already), I want you to set yourself a *realistic* target for your first step towards becoming slimmer and fitter. It's important to choose a target that's not over-ambitious to begin with so that you will be sure to succeed. Remember, after doing my seven-day plan, if you exercise and follow my advice for a healthy eating plan the rest of the time, you will continue to shape up. Then you can return for a second assault on the flab if you need to.

Getting Organised

You need to be well prepared before you start the eating plan. In order to make it as easy and painless as possible, you must first of all do some research – nothing complicated, just a careful look at exactly what your eating habits are really like.

Inconvenient Foods

All too often convenience foods and calorie-rich snacks are conveniently forgotten. That's one of the problems of fast food. Nowadays, the slightest hint of a craving is very quickly and easily appeased by wolfing down a snack. Mostly, these snacks are made with a shelf life that suits supermarkets, grocers, newsagents and confectioners so that they can be kept without refrigeration or any other special storage arrangements. Unfortunately, that generally means that they have been processed and refined so much that they lose all or most of their nutrients leaving only sugar or salt, and calories. What's worse for us is that, stripped of fibre and any bulk, the sugary snacks don't sate your hunger for long. In fact, as you have no doubt noticed, they tend to make you want another. Salty savoury snacks like nuts, cheese biscuits or other bar food make your body dehydrated and make you more thirsty. Alcohol is high in calories and low in nutrients and won't help to make you feel better. Even if you drink soft drinks instead of alcohol, you will probably consume the same amount of calories and, what's more, the extra salt in your body will take up extra water making you heavier.

That's why there are no processed or refined food products allowed in my seven-day eating plan.

Make a Food Diary

Before you start the plan, keep a diary of every single thing that passes your lips for one week. Don't be tempted to cheat or overlook anything. Look out, especially, for all those nibbles in the afternoon and early evening. Research has shown that this is often the worst time of the day for unnecessary eating. Many overweight people eat normal-sized meals at lunch and supper time but then eat as much as a good-sized meal in the form of snacks and nibbles around the late afternoon.

I don't like counting calories all the time – it just makes eating less of a pleasure and more of a chore – but it is worth taking a hard look at the calories you consume over a week. There are plenty of books available that will tell you the calorific value of most foods – you may even have one already if, like me, you've tried lots of diets before now. See if you don't find that most of your high calorie intake is in the form of snacks or alcohol. All of us can enjoy the occasional confection or social drink but very few of us can afford to take a large portion of our energy requirements in that form on a regular basis. If you do, your body will not be getting enough of the important nutrients it needs, protein, minerals, vitamins and fibre. The result is either you eat more in order to maintain an adequate level of nutrition, or you will start to redistribute valuable nutrients from within your body. In practice, this means losing muscle and gaining fat.

Once you have a better understanding of your present eating habits you can use that information to pick the best time to start my seven-day eating plan.

Tips for Starting

* If you find you eat more food at the weekends, perhaps socially as a family, don't start at the weekend.
* If it's the snacks at the office that bother you most, then do start at the weekend when you're free from the temptation.
* A useful tip for women is not to start in your premenstrual week. That's often a time when our will power is at its lowest ebb and there's a strong temptation to binge. It's also a time when a lot of women retain fluid, sometimes as much as seven pounds, so it's not a good idea to be measuring weight loss just then.
* A good strategy must take account of the psychology behind eating. Much of the excess food we eat is not in response to hunger but simply as a form of comfort. Find other ways to feel comfortable and occupy your mind.
* One of the best ways to ease your way through

the seven days is to do the eating plan with someone else, or better still, do it with a group of friends. That way you can still eat socially without having to eat separate food.

* One thing that helps a great many people to stick to their decision to lose weight is a contract. So, if you haven't already, turn to the contract on page 6, fill in the dates, find someone to witness it and sign it yourself.

* If your principles will allow it, make a bet with a friend that you'll lose the weight.

* Of course, if your partner also needs to lose weight, why don't you go on the plan together? If you can share the week you will be able to jolly each other along and help out in moments of weakness.

* Remember to keep that tight pair of jeans in a prominent place to act as an inspiration for when you're at your lowest ebb.

* Even if your partner, friends or office colleagues don't join you on the seven-day plan be sure to tell them that you are doing it. Ask them to help by not trying to persuade you to eat what you mustn't or tempt you to join them on any binges.

* There's no doubt that the evenings are the hardest part of the day when you're watching your food consumption, so be well prepared for every single evening. Warn friends and family alike that you will be pretty well booked up for seven evenings.

* Even after doing your exercises and having

19

your treat of the day, you will probably have some time on your hands, so take advantage of it and plan in advance what you will do. Go to the cinema to see a movie you've been meaning to catch for ages, simply settle down to watch a favourite programme you keep on missing on the box. But why not make a list of all the odd jobs you've been meaning to do around the house – not chores but little things you never seem to have time to do? And do them!

Succeed with the Seven-day Plan

Dieting and the Family

If you have to cook for the family it shouldn't be difficult to overlap their food with yours. Everything on the seven-day plan is highly nutritious and it will do them a power of good to eat plenty of fresh fruit and vegetables. If you have children who 'don't like greens' don't despair but also don't expect them to become converts to healthy eating overnight. Both the seven-day eating plan and my guidelines for healthy eating for the rest of your life (pages 89–156) feature lots of food in its natural state. That means much more fibre in your diet and quite a lot more bulk. Children need to be allowed time to adjust to it and I suggest you take it step by step, little by little. I promise you it will be worth it, especially if your children eat a lot of junk food at present. Junk food tends to encourage extremes of mood as the blood sugar level goes from high to low. As your children are converted to less processed food, so you may notice their moods don't fluctuate quite so dramatically. This is because they're getting a much steadier supply of energy – a natural slow release system – and they will be getting a more reliable supply of all the nutrients they need.

Reasons to Succeed

When you go on my seven-day plan, not only will you lose weight, but you will feel better and, most important, you will be *in control*. For me, fat equals miserable and one of the reasons we're all so miserable when we're overweight is that we feel out of control. Once you get your eating under control, you'll feel much, much happier not only about food but about yourself.

* You'll stop being obsessed by food.
* Your self-image will improve.
* You'll gain confidence.
* The knowledge that you'll never be fat again will give you a new lease of life.

So, believe me, it's worth it. Make the effort for yourself and no one else. You're important – give yourself the highest priority.

Relaxation

Every evening of the seven-day plan, I want you to do some simple yoga exercises. These are not specifically to tone up muscles but more to help you to become in tune with your body and by doing so become more relaxed. Don't attempt too much at first but as the exercises become easier, do more of them until you have a daily routine which incorporates them all.

To start, try yoga breathing. First of all you take a deep breath in through your nose to the count of four. When you think you've got all the air you can into your lungs take in another little sharp sniff, and then relax and breathe out through your mouth. Keep exhaling until you feel empty then a little extra to squeeze that last breath out. Feel yourself relaxing each time you breathe out. Feel that oxygen filling up your lungs and feel it flowing round your body. Do that at least five times when you are ready for bed and do it anywhere, inside or out, standing, sitting or lying, when you want to feel more relaxed.

Next, build on your yoga breathing routine with some deep muscle relaxation and positive imagery. Find a quiet place that's comfortable, like the bedroom and lie down and close your eyes. Concentrate on your right hand if you are right-handed and your left if you are left-handed. Make as tight a fist as you can and then relax. That makes you aware how relaxed you want to be. Now concentrate on making your hand feel warm and heavy. Repeat it to yourself: warm and heavy. Let your whole arm become warm and heavy. Then let the arm go and feel it sink into the bed. Now repeat the exercise for your right or left foot and feel your lower leg and then your thigh become warm and heavy. Carry the sensation up into your pelvis and abdomen, letting them all sink into the bed. Now on to your chest and finally your jaw, neck and mouth. End up by telling your forehead to be cool, cool, cool.

If you haven't done yoga before, don't expect to master it in one go and don't rush it. Practise this routine for fifteen or twenty minutes every day if you can; even a few minutes, if that's all the time you can make, is better than nothing. Remember to find a quiet and comfortable place without distractions and start with the yoga breathing.

After you have mastered the deep muscle relaxation exercises, try some mental relaxation. Mental relaxation will help you combat stressful thoughts and worries and, with positive imagery, will help you to take control of your body. As before, start with some yoga breathing then the next thing I want you to do is some free association. Let your mind flit from one thought to another. Think of something positive and pleasant and just follow a line of thought wherever it takes you. If an unpleasant thought comes into your head say NO and keep it out. The colour blue is the most relaxing colour. Think of a blue sky and a blue sea. Then think about your breathing, feel the air filling your lungs and then breathe out slowly and relax.

Make time each day for these relaxation techniques and you will find that you are less bothered by stress and worry.

Food for the Seven-day Plan

There are several dishes that you will be eating quite regularly when you do the seven-day plan because they are the dieter's best friends. They are satisfying and they depress the appetite and suppress cravings. Some of them are best made in advance, others may not be familiar to you. Here are the basic recipes and some serving suggestions.

Porridge

Porridge is my favourite breakfast. It sets you up for the rest of the day, it's nutritious and it does you a power of good. Oats, and especially oat bran, are one of the richest sources of soluble fibre. Research has shown that regular daily helpings of oats in one form or another can actually reduce the level of cholesterol and other low-density lipoproteins in our blood – over and above the effect of any special low-fat diet. Furthermore, the sticky sponge-like mass of soluble fibre slows down the rate of absorption of carbohydrates and helps to even out the tendency for the blood glucose level to shoot up and down. A steadier level of blood glucose means you will feel better and are less likely to get cravings.

For one person

* Take half a cupful of oats (about 50 g/2 oz).
* Add about 1 ¼ cups of water.
* Use a good pinch of salt to taste.
* Bring to the boil so it begins to bubble, and then simmer for 3 minutes, stirring all the time.
* Serve with up to 150 ml/¼ pint skimmed milk.

As a general rule, I don't think you should add salt to food but I like a little with my porridge. If you aren't bothered then don't! Many people have more difficulty eating porridge without lashings of sugar or spoonfuls of syrup. I'm afraid that is absolutely out of the question. If you like it sweet, you could use a low-calorie sweetener but, better still, use an unprocessed sweetener – fruit. A heaped tablespoonful of chopped dried fruit – apricots, raisins, prunes – is delicious. Alternatively, chop in a fresh peach or nectarine. Either way your porridge tastes sweeter without resorting to processed and refined foodstuffs.

Rice

Rice is one of the foods I recommend for the early evening meal. It's a good, nutritious source of energy in the right form – unprocessed carbohydrate. Make sure you buy wholegrain rice – that's mostly sold as brown rice. White rice has had the husk removed and has then been polished, losing most of its goodness.

To Cook Wholegrain Rice

* It helps to begin by dry frying or cracking it in a pan. You don't need any oil: just heat the pan, add the rice and stir. After a minute or so the rice will start to crack and jump about; stir more vigorously so that it doesn't burn.
* Once most of it is cracked, pour in the water. Now recipes vary wildly in the amount of water they recommend. You can simply use a lot, and then drain the rice when it's ready. That's probably the easiest way if you are using a hob.
* Some people prefer to cook rice with only one and a quarter times as much water. Add boiled water from the kettle and give it a good stir. Once the water has returned to the boil, stop stirring and leave it alone from now on. Put a lid on it and place it in the oven for about 45 minutes at gas mark 5/190°C/375°F until all the water is absorbed and the rice is cooked.

Be adventurous and add seasoning to the rice:

* You can start by adding half a finely chopped onion to the water and using a teaspoonful of black pepper and black cumin.
* One or two squashed cardamoms and a little ground turmeric will give it an authentic Indian flavour and colour.
* If you like a nutty flavour, spoil yourself by adding 25 g/1 oz wild rice to 225 g/8 oz wholegrain rice. The black seeds are really grass seed not rice at all but they make the dish look and taste rather exotic.
* Another way to make it special is to buy a little real saffron, not turmeric, the yellow spice which is sometimes confusingly called saffron, but the tiny red stamens picked from the hearts of crocuses. A good pinch in the rice while it's cooking and a little more added just before serving gives a wonderful colour and aroma.

Once it's cooked and cooled, keep the rice in an airtight container in the fridge, ready for your six o'clock mealtimes.

Dahl

Dahl is another excellent food which I recommend for your six o'clock meal. Again, once it is prepared, it can be kept in the fridge and you can eat a little with rice or on its own. If you've never heard of it, you have a treat in store. It's made from split peas or lentils and it's very nutritious. Like all the pulses, it is rich in protein and fibre but low in fat – just what we want.

To Cook Dahl

225 g/8 oz split peas/lentils
300 ml/½ pint water
1 small onion
1 clove garlic
cumin
black pepper

* Start by soaking the lentils overnight.
* The next day, rinse them thoroughly, add the water and boil briskly for 10 minutes.
* Then reduce the heat, add the finely sliced onion and garlic and simmer until the lentils are cooked and the water absorbed. Depending on how fresh they are, that could be 30 or as much as 45 minutes.
* Don't add any salt. Not just because we are cutting down, but also because it makes the lentils tougher.
* Season with generous amounts of cumin and black pepper. As a variation, try turmeric and cloves, or make a hot version with some fresh chillis. Don't be afraid to add quite a lot of spice – lentils need strong flavouring for best results.

Once the lentils are cooked, stir well and you should have a delicious paste with the consistency of pease pudding (which is also a food I highly recommend).

If you can't wait overnight, here's a quick way to make dahl:

* Pour 1.25 litres/2 pints of boiling water over the lentils and let stand for 1 hour.
* Drain and rinse thoroughly.
* Cook at high pressure in a pressure cooker for 15 minutes.
* Continue the simmering and add the seasoning on a hob, stirring frequently.

Stock

Stock is the secret to making delicious soups, sauces and many other meals. It's very simple to prepare and you can make it using animal bones or just vegetables. If you have salad vegetables that are slightly past their best (but not bruised or bad) this is an excellent use for them. Also, any foliage from fennel, celery or young carrots adds to the flavour. Be sure to keep the stalks when washing and preparing parsley and other herbs – they contain most of the flavour.

* Clean vegetables and trim off any bruised parts.

* Put your stock bones in a large pot, the larger the better.
* Cover with plenty of water (about 2 litres/3½ pints).
* Add 1 or 2 chopped carrots for sweetness.
* Add 1 or 2 onions or leeks, or any member of the onion family except garlic.
* Add celery, fennel or any similar salad vegetables as you choose.
* Season with 1 or 2 fresh bay leaves, 12 peppercorns, a sprig of fresh thyme, perhaps a little rosemary, and great handfuls of parsley.
* Bring to the boil and simmer for about 2 hours.
* Strain off the bones and vegetables and discard. Return the liquor to the pan and reduce down to about 600 ml/1 pint in volume. Don't forget it, put a timer on and keep checking.
* If you have used bones, the stock should now be quite thick. Remove from the heat and leave to cool.
* After cooling, or sitting in the fridge overnight, all the fat will have solidified as a white layer on top that can be easily removed. What's left underneath is a wonderfully tasty and nutritious jelly of stock suitable for making soups, gravies or adding to any dish that uses liquid.
* A good way to store stock is to freeze it. If you are going to do this, pour into suitable freezer containers before it has cooled and remove the fat later.

If you don't want to use bones, you can still make a delicious sweet stock with vegetables and herbs. Don't bother to reduce it as it is not going to form a jelly and prolonged boiling will remove some of the goodness. Instead, start with less water, perhaps 1.25 litres/2 pints depending on the size of the pot and the amount of vegetables. Incidentally, chefs call this a *court bouillon* and it is an excellent poaching medium for fish.

If you have a pressure cooker, you can make stock in about 40 minutes, or 20 minutes if it is without bones.

Soups

Once you have made your stock, it can be quickly transformed into a highly nutritious soup. All the soups in my eating plan are potato based, and for good reason. Potatoes supply lots of carbohydrate and lots of fibre. Leave the skins on because that's also where all the minerals and vitamins are. My recipe couldn't be simpler:

* Place stock in pan.
* Add 1 or 2 chopped, washed and scrubbed potatoes.
* Add 1 chopped medium-sized onion.
* Add other ingredients as appropriate (see below).
* Simmer for 20–30 minutes.
* Liquidise if you want to make it thick and creamy.

Suggestions for Other Ingredients

* Carrot (2 diced or grated) and fresh coriander leaves.
* Leeks (2 or 3, omit onion) 1 bay leaf and lots of parsley.
* 225 g/8 oz frozen peas and fresh mint.
* 175 g/6 oz brown lentils, 2 sticks of celery, black pepper and 1 teaspoon crushed coriander seeds.
* 125 g/4 oz grated cooked beetroot, seasoned with 1 teaspoon ground cumin.
* 50 g/2 oz each of peas, carrots, cauliflower, leek, swede, all diced (also dice potato and onion), black pepper and parsley.

Salads

I've put the salads into a special section because you can use them as a meal any time. They are particularly nutritious and very filling, so any one of them will keep you going for a good two hours.

Mixed Salads

These can be made with any amount of the following:

bean sprouts
carrot
celery
chicory
cress
cucumber
endive
assorted lettuce leaves
green/red peppers

radicchio
radish
raw spinach
spring onion
tomato

Dress with a little (2 teaspoons) of French
    dressing
or 2 tablespoons of very low-fat natural
    yoghurt dressing (see recipe opposite)
or 2 tablespoons of rice vinegar.

Broccoli Salad (serves two)

450 g/1 lb broccoli, trimmed
2 sweet red peppers
Sauce
1 clove garlic
½ tablespoon sunflower oil
225 g/8 oz tomatoes, chopped
pepper

Cook the broccoli until just tender, rinse with cold
water and drain well.

Cut the broccoli lengthways into smaller pieces.
Grill the red peppers, turning them as they brown.
Wrap them in a clean cloth and allow them to cool
for 10 minutes. Peel off the wrinkled skin and slice
the peppers into thin strips, removing the seeds
and the inner membranes.

Cook the crushed garlic in the oil until just beginning to brown, add the chopped tomatoes and

season with pepper. Simmer gently for 5 minutes or so. Remove from the heat and liquidise, process or press through a sieve. Arrange the broccoli in a flat serving dish, pour the sauce over it and arrange the strips of red peppers round the edge. Allow to cool.

Yoghurt Dressing

150g/5 oz very low fat natural yoghurt
1 coffeespoon freshly ground black pepper or nutmeg or cumin
1 desertspoon raspberry vinegar (ordinary wine vinegar will do)
1 tablespoon parsley/chives/leaf coriander
1 clove garlic, crushed
1 tablespoon pine nuts or sesame seeds

Place all ingredients in a screw-top jar and shake firmly. Will store in the refrigerator for up to two days.

Shopping Checklist

Use this checklist when you go shopping. But first plan at least the first few days of your seven-day eating plan and look at the specific ingredients for those dishes. Don't buy more than you need. Remember, fresh fish and offal are best eaten the day they are bought.

Fish/Meat (showing approximate portion size)

50 g/2 oz anchovies in brine
small herring or mackerel
medium-sized kipper
125 g/4 oz monkfish
150 g/5 oz salmon cutlet
125 g/4 oz smoked salmon
175 g/6 oz seafood (mussels, prawns, scallops, crab)

175 g/6 oz trout
125 g/4 oz tuna in brine
175 g/6 oz white fish (cod, haddock, coley, hake, plaice, sole, turbot)

125 g/4 oz calves' or lambs' liver
150 g/5 oz chicken breasts
75 g/3 oz boneless chicken
50 g/2 oz chicken livers
chicken/turkey bones for stock
175 g/6 oz rabbit, diced and boned
225 g/8 oz turkey breast fillet
125 g/4 oz smoked turkey

Staples

beans, dried (aduki, chick peas, green flageolet, haricot, kidney)
lentils/split peas
porridge
wholegrain (brown) rice
wild rice

Dairy

cottage cheese
goat's or ewe's milk cheese
low-fat cheese
eggs, up to 2 size 4
milk, skimmed
very low-fat natural yoghurt

Vegetables

asparagus
aubergine
French beans
baby beetroots
broccoli
cabbage
carrots
cauliflower
celeriac
courgettes
garlic
leeks
mangetout
okra
onions
parsnips
frozen peas/sweetcorn
potatoes, good baking and boiling
spinach
baby sweetcorn

Salad Vegetables

bean sprouts
celery
chicory
cucumber
fennel
lettuce

green/red peppers
radish
spring onions
watercress
other salad leaves to choice (e.g. endive,
  radicchio)

Fruit

apples
apricots
bananas
berries (e.g. strawberries, raspberries,
  blueberries)
dried soaked fruit (e.g. apricots, prunes)
grapefruit
lemons/limes
mango
melon
nectarines
oranges
papaya
peaches
pears
pineapple
tomatoes
other exotic fruit (e.g. guava, passion fruit)

Seasonings

basil
bay leaves
chilli pepper, red
chilli powder
chives
Chinese five spice
coriander leaves
coriander seeds
cumin
fennel seeds
fresh root ginger
marjoram
mint
mustard seed
nutmeg
parsley
pepper, black
saffron
sage
tarragon
thyme
turmeric

Condiments and Other Groceries

herb teas
mustard (any as preferred)
oil (grapeseed/sunflower/safflower) for
   cooking and dressing

oil (olive/walnut/sesame) for flavouring –
   used in small amounts
tomato juice
tomato purée
Tabasco
vinegar (wine/rice/raspberry)
walnuts/hazelnuts

Friendly Foods

carrots
celery
chicory
coffee
cucumber
low-calorie drinks
green/red peppers
radish
spring onions
tea
small whole tomatoes

One a Day Snacks

If you are still hungry after eating the six meals in
the eating plan you may eat one of the following
once in a day:

up to 24 berries
1 slice of pineapple

1 whole fruit
1 boiled potato
8 peeled prawns
1 slice of smoked salmon
1 very low-fat natural yoghurt
½ cup of soup
1 small jelly
1 glass of tomato juice

Banned Foods

The following foods are strictly off limits for the duration of the seven-day eating plan:

avocados
fried foods
any red meat
any refined or processed foods
any sauces, chutneys, pickles
all kinds of sugar, sweets and any jam, marmalade or spread
any tinned foods in oil, syrup or sauce
any wheat, maize, rye, barley produce including breakfast cereals, biscuits, cakes

The Seven-day Eating Plan

Each day, for the next seven days, I want you to stick only to the foods on the checklist. It is important to eat all six meals in order to keep your metabolism working in a high gear. Try to space them so that you don't go more than two and a half hours without eating. To make it easy I have provided menu suggestions for each meal throughout the week and alternatives in case there is something you don't like. Once you have done the initial preparation for the six o'clock meals (e.g. rice, dahl, soups), only the lunch and dinner menus require any time and, depending on your situation, you may prefer to select quick and easy meals.

Make sure you drink at least two pints of still water through each day. Try to take a glass with every meal.

Breakfast

For breakfast each day I really do recommend porridge, but if you would like a change, you can have up to two size 4 eggs in the week – either boiled or for lunch as an omelette. Similarly, you can ring the changes with the occasional kipper for breakfast. Make sure you have a piece of fruit as well.

Mid-morning

For your mid-morning food I suggest another piece of fresh fruit – it needn't be simply another apple if you take the trouble to stock up on some more unusual fruits before you start. If you like it, a little goat's or ewe's milk cheese (about 25 g/1 oz) works particularly well as an accompaniment to, for example, pears. A rice cake is another good idea, or a low-fat yoghurt.

Lunch

The lunch menus are designed to cater for the office worker as well as those of you who work at home. Many of the meals can be packaged easily so that they can travel with you. Others are more elaborate and might be more suitable for the weekend. All of them are quite appetising enough to serve to the family or even to guests. As well as the main course dish, have a dessert of fruit – perhaps some berries or slice of pineapple or choose from your fruit bowl as seems appropriate – and drink plenty of water.

Mid-afternoon

My family is rather fond of home-made oat (if not already done) biscuits. They're not oatcakes. You make them with very little fat and no sugar and they're delicious (see recipe on page 51). I suggest you have one of these, or a very low-fat yoghurt or some more fruit for your mid-afternoon meal.

Early Evening Meal

This is the time that most of us eat those high calorie nibbles that put on the weight. That's why it's so important to be well prepared with the right food for this meal, unprocessed carbohydrate in the form of hot soup or three or four tablespoons of rice or dahl or a mixture of both.

Dinner

I have given dinner recipes in quantities for two servings but if you are eating alone just halve the ingredients! However, if you are eating with a partner or friend don't let them dismiss the menu out of hand. I think you'll find they are surprised by how tasty the meals on the eating plan are. As for lunch, choose your dessert from the fruit bowl and remember to drink plenty of still water.

Day 1

Breakfast

Try porridge with sliced apricots today.

Mid-morning

Half a papaya with a squeeze of lemon or lime juice.

Lunch

Marinated White Fish ✗

175 g/6 oz fillet white fish
3 teaspoons lemon or lime juice
½ teaspoon fennel seeds, crushed
¼ red chilli, chopped

Place all the ingredients in a dish and marinate overnight in the fridge – no cooking necessary! Serve with a mixed salad tossed in 1 teaspoon French dressing.

Alternative Lunch

Orange and Kidney Bean Salad ✓

75 g/3 oz cooked kidney beans
1 large orange, peeled and cut into segments
2 sticks of celery, chopped
1 tablespoon French dressing made with whole-grain mustard and dash of lemon juice
large handful iceberg lettuce
50 g/2 oz hard goat's or ewe's milk cheese

Mix the beans, orange and celery with the dressing and pile on to a bed of lettuce. Scatter slices of cheese over.

Mid-afternoon

One plain oat biscuit (see recipe below) or half a mango with lemon juice.

Plain Oat Biscuits (makes about 20)

175 g/6 oz oatmeal
50 g/2 oz rolled oats
pinch of bicarbonate of soda
50 g/2 oz margarine
1 egg yolk

Mix together the dry ingredients. Rub in the margarine until the mixture resembles dry breadcrumbs. Add the egg yolk and mix to a firm dough, then knead lightly. Roll out to a thickness of about .6 mm (¼ inch) and cut into shapes and transfer to a greased baking tray. Bake for about 15 minutes or until darker in colour at gas mark 4/180°C/350°F.

Early Evening

A cup of hot soup or three or four tablespoons of rice or dahl or a mixture of both.

Dinner

Oven-poached Chicken (serves two)

2 175 g/6 oz chicken breasts
½ medium onion, sliced
175 g/6 oz each of French beans, cabbage and
    celeriac, cut into sticks
150 ml/¼ pint stock

Arrange the chicken pieces in an ovenproof dish, scatter the vegetables over them and pour in the stock. Cover and bake for 30 minutes at gas mark 5/190°C/375°F.

Alternative Dinner

Grilled Liver with Orange and Sage (serves two)

225 g/8 oz lambs' or calves' liver, thinly sliced
1 teaspoon grapeseed oil
½ orange, cut in wedges
1 tablespoon sage, chopped
black pepper

Brush the liver with oil, and grill for 2 minutes on each side under a hot grill. Squeeze the orange over, and sprinkle with the sage and pepper. Serve with 175 g/6 oz sliced cabbage, 175 g/6 oz sliced celeriac, and 175 g/6 oz French beans which have all been braised in 150 ml/¼ pint stock.

Tip of the Day

Take your food seriously. Make eating a separate and distinct part of your life, a familiar routine. In other words sit down and concentrate on your meal. Don't read the newspaper or watch the TV. Set the table. Chew your food slowly and thoroughly. Drink plenty of water with your food. Remember, your appetite control centre takes a while to switch off the hunger signals. As soon as you begin to feel full, stop. Do not stuff yourself!

Exercise of the Day

The thighs are the biggest muscles in the body so they can burn up quite a few calories if they are exercised and toned up. I want you to start your exercising by concentrating on the thighs. It couldn't be much simpler: all you have to do is stride out. Wherever you are walking, take bigger steps. Now, many women don't do nearly enough of this because they are wearing tight skirts and high heels, so switch to fuller skirts or start wearing trousers. As an extra bonus, you'll feel better, more positive and more confident.

Treat of the Day

For her: give yourself a face-pack – the whole treatment.

For him: try out that new look. Start with a hair cut or different style.

Day 2

Breakfast

As an alternative to porridge, try half a grapefruit and a grilled kipper.

Mid-morning

Fresh fruit – why not crunch on an apple?

Lunch

Bean Salad

175 g/6 oz cooked weight of mixed dried beans, soaked overnight and cooked until tender
¼ cucumber, diced
1 heaped teaspoon chopped onion

Dressing
150 ml/¼ pint very low-fat yoghurt
dash of lemon juice
2 teaspoons parsley/chives, chopped

Drain the beans thoroughly and put in a serving dish. Add the cucumber and onion. Mix together the dressing ingredients and pour over the salad, tossing well.

Alternative Lunch

125 g/4 oz cooked chicken (skin removed before cooking) or 125 /4 oz smoked salmon or trout served with a mixed salad.

Mid-afternoon

Have another oat biscuit or a banana.

Early Evening

If you would prefer, drink a cool glass of tomato juice instead of hot soup.

Dinner

Stir-fried Turkey Breast (serves two) ✓

2 teaspoons sesame oil
225 g/8 oz turkey breast fillet, cut into thin strips,
   no fat
125 g/4 oz mangetout
125 g/4 oz fennel, sliced
pinch of Chinese five spice

Heat the oil in a wok or frying pan and fry the
turkey strips quickly over a high heat. Add the
vegetables and spice and stir continuously for
another couple of minutes, so that the vegetables
are still crunchy. Serve with 225 g/8 oz baby
sweetcorn, boiled, peeled and scattered with
chopped spring onion.

Alternative Dinner

Steamed mussels (serves two)

700 g/1½ lb fresh mussels
150 ml/¼ pint vegetable or fish stock
1 onion, finely chopped
125 g/4 oz bean sprouts
125 g/4 oz mangetout
125 g/4 oz French beans
1 heaped tablespoon parsley, chopped

Clean and debeard the mussels, discarding any that are not firmly shut. Bring the stock and onion to a fierce boil and add the mussels. Cover and simmer for 3 minutes, giving the pan an occasional shake. Remove from the heat and allow to stand for another 2 minutes. Remove the mussels from the pot, reject any that have not opened, and keep warm. Cook the vegetables together in the mussel liquor. Serve the mussels and vegetables garnished with parsley.

Tip of the Day

Treat meat as a condiment. Try to have four times as many vegetables as meat on your plate. Start with the vegetables and leave some meat if you begin to feel full. When you have finished the seven-day plan, try not to eat red meat more than once a week. Try extending the meat or mince in meat pies and casseroles with the addition of some plant protein like lentils or haricot beans, which make up the core of many well-known meat dishes, such as cassoulet from the south of France.

Exercise of the Day

From now on I want you to ignore lifts and escalators wherever possible. Take the stairs. Don't rush into this if you are fairly unfit – start by walking up, step by step, and hold on to the handrail. As you feel fitter, start walking up without using the hand-rail. Then take two steps at a time, using the hand-rail. Then do two steps at a time without the help of the handrail. When you've mastered that and feel reasonably comfortable, run up the stairs, or esca-lators, two at a time! It's exercising those thighs and it's good for your heart as well.

Treat of the Day

For her: condition and treat your hair as you've been promising yourself for months.

For him: treat yourself to a relaxing sauna and massage.

Day 3

Breakfast

Porridge sweetened with some sliced prunes.

Mid-morning

Tangerine.

Lunch

Cottage Cheese and Walnut Salad

Large handful of endive
½ apple, sliced
½ onion, sliced
½ head of chicory
125 g/4 oz low-fat cottage cheese
1 tablespoon broken walnuts
1 teaspoon mint
½ teaspoon walnut oil

Arrange the endive, apple and onion slices, chicory and cottage cheese attractively on a plate. Scatter with the walnuts and mint and trickle the oil over.

Alternative Lunch

Mexican Green Beans

1 teaspoon sesame oil
175 g/6 oz haricots verts (or any green beans)
½ red pepper, sliced
½ small onion, sliced
3 tablespoons stock
½ teaspoon tomato purée
pinch of chilli powder
or 1 sliced and deseeded fresh green chilli

Heat the oil in a pan and stir-fry the vegetables for a couple of minutes. Add the stock, tomato purée and chilli powder and simmer until liquid is absorbed. Serve with 50 g/2 oz cooked whole-grain rice.

Mid-afternoon

A tomato.

Early Evening

A cup of soup of your choice, or a cold jacket potato.

Dinner

Rabbit Casserole (serves two)

350 g/12 oz cubed boned rabbit
1 clove garlic, crushed
2 sticks celery, chopped
225 g/8 oz carrot, chopped
1 medium onion, sliced
300 ml/½ pint chicken stock
1 teaspoon French mustard
1 teaspoon tarragon
black pepper

Arrange the rabbit in a casserole dish and add all the other ingredients. Cover and cook for about 1½ hours at gas mark 5/190°C/375°F. Serve with 225 g/8 oz asparagus and leeks, each lightly boiled.

Alternative Dinner

Ratatouille (225 g/8 oz approx cooked weight per portion)

450 g/1 lb tomatoes, quartered
1 medium aubergine, diced
2 courgettes, sliced
1 onion, sliced
1 green pepper, sliced
50 g/2 oz chick peas, soaked overnight
1 clove garlic, crushed
1 teaspoon dried marjoram
300 ml/½ pint tomato juice

Simmer all the ingredients gently in a pan until the chick peas are tender (about 1 hour). Serve with 25 g/1 oz grated Edam on each portion.

Tip of the Day

If you feel hungry and have the urge to buy a snack on impulse, try to allay that feeling by positive imagery. Think of what that fatty or sugary snack will end up as in your body – perhaps another few grammes of fat! It may not be a genuine hunger at all, if you are sticking to my plan and eating six times a day; it could simply be a need for some oral gratification in much the same way as cigarette smoking can be. However, if you really are hungry, eat some carbohydrate – but make certain it is

unprocessed carbohydrate. Eat something like a
banana or half a jacket potato (or some rice or dahl
or soup if you are at home). Half an hour after
eating the hunger will go.

Exercise of the Day

This exercise is designed to improve your tummy
muscles and has a great effect on your waistline as
well. It can be quite difficult to begin with but it
soon becomes easy if you persist. I want you to pull
your tummy right in ten times. As that becomes
easier, try holding it in for five seconds each time.
Now, this is a terribly simple exercise and you can
do it anywhere, sitting at a desk, standing in a bus
queue or even while you are walking, so make a
point of doing it whenever you can. You'll be
amazed at the results.

Treat of the Day

For her: give yourself a complete home manicure
with polish in a new colour.

For him: try out a different look, and pat yourself
on the back with some new items to add to your
wardrobe.

Day 4

Breakfast

If you would like a change from porridge, I suggest one poached egg out of your week's quota accompanied by an orange.

Mid-morning

A nectarine, if in season, or a slice of pineapple.

Lunch

Salad Niçoise

handful of crisp lettuce
¼ green pepper, sliced
50 g/2 oz French beans, cooked
1 stick of celery, chopped
1 tomato, sliced
1 tablespoon onion, sliced
125 g/4 oz tuna fish in brine, well drained
2 anchovy fillets, desalted overnight in milk

French dressing
3 teaspoons grapeseed oil
1 teaspoon olive or other strong-flavoured oil
1 tablespoon lemon juice
1 teaspoon wine vinegar
½ teaspoon mustard
black pepper

Line a bowl with the lettuce and layer the vegetables on top, finishing with the tuna fish and anchovy fillets. Make the dressing in a screwtop jar, shake well and pour over the salad.

Alternative Lunch

Turkey Coleslaw

125 g/4 oz cooked or smoked turkey cut into strips
50 g/2 oz cabbage, shredded
1 carrot, grated
1 teaspoon grated onion
15 g/½ oz dried, soaked apricot, chopped
1 tablespoon broken hazelnuts
black pepper
2 tablespoons yoghurt dressing (see page 37)

Mix together all the ingredients, toss well in the dressing and serve in a bowl.

Mid-afternoon

An apple.

Early Evening

One helping of dahl.

Dinner

Tandoori Chicken and Spicy Vegetables (serves two)

2 chicken breast fillets (about 125 g/4 oz)

Marinade

juice of 1 lemon
150 ml/¼ pint very low-fat natural yoghurt
1 teaspoon tomato purée
1 clove garlic, crushed
pinch each of ground chilli, coriander, cumin,
   ginger and pepper

Spicy vegetables
2 teaspoons sesame oil
125 g/4 oz baby new potatoes, parboiled
125 g/4 oz okra or aubergine
175 g/6 oz cauliflower florets
125 g/4 oz courgettes, cut into sticks
2 tablespoons chicken stock
½ teaspoon cumin seed
½ teaspoon black mustard seed

Marinate the chicken in the lemon juice for 10 minutes then add the yoghurt, tomato purée, garlic and seasoning and leave for at least 2 hours or overnight. Cook under a fierce grill for about 10 minutes, turning once and basting occasionally (line the grill tray with foil to make cleaning easy). While the chicken is cooking, heat the oil in a large pan and stir-fry the prepared vegetables. Add the stock and seeds and serve once liquid is absorbed.

Alternative Dinner

Lentil and Potato Pie (serves two)

125 g/4 oz brown lentils (presoaked)
225 g/8 oz carrots, chopped
1 medium onion, sliced
1 clove garlic, crushed
300 ml/½ pint stock
pinch of marjoram
black pepper
225 g/8 oz potato, mashed
1 tablespoon low-fat yoghurt
1 tablespoon spring onion, chopped

Simmer the lentils and vegetables in the stock until tender (about 45 minutes). Drain well, season with marjoram and pepper and place in a pie dish. Cover with mashed potatoes, creamed with the yoghurt and sprinkle with spring onions.

Tip of the Day

If you eat salty food, your body takes up more water, which adds to your weight and alters your shape. Eat less salt and avoid fattening salted snacks. Instead, try to eat more natural diuretics – that is, foods that help you lose water. If you drink plenty of still water every day of the eating plan and keep natural diuretics on the menu, you will lose more weight. The most easily available plant diuretics are:

* Parsley – a wonderful herb in its own right but also a very handy alternative to salt as a seasoning.
* Capsicums – that's red, green or yellow peppers. They are also very rich in vitamin C (they have even more than citrus fruit).
* Asparagus – a delicious treat and a very powerful diuretic. You may notice this before the end of a meal!
* Real coffee – a cup of this in the morning if you like it, but don't overdo it.

Exercise of the Day

This exercise is for your pelvic floor muscles and is especially important for women who have had children. It can stop you from developing incontinence in later life, or even a prolapse – both of which are fairly common. The easiest way to learn how to contract these muscles is to try and stop the flow of urine next time you go to the loo. Those muscles in your groin that you are exercising, when you succeed, are your pelvic floor muscles. Don't worry if it seems difficult at first, that's quite normal and it's probably because they've been neglected for a long time. Keep practising each time you go to the loo and eventually you will know how to do it anywhere, anytime. One added bonus of this exercise is it can improve your sexual enjoyment.

Treat of the Day

For her: what about a home pedicure so your feet can keep up with your fingers? Deal with that rough skin with a removing cream and polish your toenails.

For him: why not join a swish gym or health club as your next step towards a slimmer and fitter existence?

Day 5

Breakfast

Brown Rice Breakfast Dish

125 g/4 oz cooked, short grain brown rice
100 ml/4 fl oz water or water and juice of soaked,
   dried fruit

Optional ingredients
sesame, sunflower seed or almond meal
25 g/1 oz finely grated carrot
25 g/1 oz fruit purée (apricot, apple, pear)
1 teaspoon light tahini

Combine ingredients of choice in a saucepan, omitting fruit purée if used. Stir over medium heat, bring to the boil then reduce heat, cover and simmer for 5 minutes. Tahini gives a creamy texture and flavour. Add fruit purée, if used, before serving.

Mid-morning

24 (½ cup) blackberries, blueberries or raspberries.

Lunch

Seafood Salad

175 g/6 oz mixed steamed seafood made with mussels, clams, prawns, scallops, crab
1 small carrot cut into ribbons with vegetable
   peeler
1 spring onion, shredded
lemon juice and olive oil to moisten

Scatter the carrot and onion over the seafood and
flavour sparingly with the lemon juice and olive oil.

Alternative Lunch

65 g/2½ oz smoked mackerel or an omelette using
the two size 4 eggs out of your week's quota (only
wipe the pan with oil), served with a mixed salad.

Mid-afternoon

A pear with, if you like, a slice of goat's or ewe's
milk cheese.

Early Evening

Rice and dahl or one very low-fat yoghurt.

Dinner

Stuffed Peppers/Tomatoes/Aubergines

1 or 2 green peppers or large tomatoes or
  1 aubergine for each person

Stuffing
225 g/8 oz cooked brown rice
75 g/3 oz frozen peas and sweetcorn
½ small onion, finely chopped
1 heaped tablespoon mixed fresh herbs, chopped
black pepper
150 ml/¼ pint tomato juice

Prepare the vegetables to be stuffed by hollowing
out the insides. Mix together all the stuffing ingredients moistening with the tomato juice, and pile
into the vegetable shells. Arrange in an ovenproof
dish and pour in enough water to cover the base.
Cover and bake for 45 minutes to 1 hour at gas
mark 5/190°C/375°F.

Alternative Dinner

Vegetable Hotpot (serves two)

2 teaspoons grapeseed oil
1 onion, sliced
1 medium aubergine, diced
2 courgettes, sliced
½ cauliflower, cut into florets
1 teaspoon tomato purée
150 ml/¼ pint stock
1 teaspoon dried basil
Tabasco and black pepper to taste
350 g/12 oz potato, sliced
1 tablespoon grated parmesan

Heat 1 teaspoon of oil in an ovenproof casserole, add the onion, aubergine, courgettes and cauliflower and fry for 2 minutes. Add the tomato purée, stock, basil seasoning and bring to the boil. Arrange the sliced potato on top, brush with 1 teaspoon of grapeseed oil and bake at gas mark 5/190°C/375°F for 1 hour. Ten minutes before serving, sprinkle parmesan on top.

Tip of the Day

Never let yourself get too hungry either while on the eating plan or afterwards. If you feel genuinely hungry it's much better to bring your meal forward a little rather than get ravenous with the result that you wolf down more food than you actually need. Remember, eat slowly.

Exercise of the Day

If you have been sticking to the exercise for the last four days you have probably already improved your posture but now I want you to think about it more deliberately. Don't look down as you walk around, as that way you can encourage droopy shoulders or even a dowager's hump in later life. It's bad for your breathing, your digestion and your back. Hold your head up and keep your shoulders back – though not too stiffly, this isn't the army! You should find your chest is now sticking out a bit more and the clothes around your waist become less ruckled and rumpled. What's more, your silhouette will improve and you will look more confident. One added bonus of all this is that research shows that muggers will be less inclined to pick on you because you will look and feel confident and more assertive as you stride out.

Treat of the Day

For her: experiment with that new eye make-up you saw in a magazine and are too scared to wear in public.

For him: pay some attention to those nails with a long-overdue manicure or pedicure.

Day 6

Breakfast

Porridge with apple or one boiled egg out of the week's quota with an orange.

Mid-morning

A couple of basic biscuits (see recipe below).

Basic Biscuits

175 g/6 oz mixed bean flours
25 g/1 oz oil
50–75 ml/2–3 fl oz water
25 g/1 oz sesame seed meal (optional)
2 teaspoons baking powder (optional)

Mix all the ingredients thoroughly. Drop dessert-spoonfuls on to a lightly greased baking sheet. Bake for 15 minutes at gas mark 3/160°C/325°F. Remember, just one or two at a time!

Lunch

Chicken or Monkfish Kebabs

75 g/3 oz boneless chicken
50 g/2 oz chicken livers
¼ each of green, red and yellow peppers
1 teaspoon grapeseed oil
thyme

OR

125 g/4 oz monkfish, cut into strips, marinated for
  2 hours
6 cherry tomatoes
thick slices of onion
1 teaspoon grapeseed oil

Marinade
2 teaspoons orange juice
½ teaspoon coriander seed, crushed

Arrange kebabs on skewers, alternating meat or fish and vegetables in a colourful way. Lightly brush with oil and put under a hot grill – or barbeque – for about 10 minutes, turning occasionally. Serve with a mixed salad.

Alternative Lunch

Grilled Fish with Steamed Vegetables (serves two)

225 g/8 oz white fish (cod, haddock, plaice, sole, monkfish)
1 teaspoon grapeseed oil
225 g/8 oz leeks, sliced
225 g/8 oz courgettes, sliced
225 g/8 oz French beans

Brush the fish with the oil and grill under a medium heat until cooked, turning once. Meanwhile steam the vegetables. Serve with wedges of lemon or lime.

Mid-afternoon

A cup of home-made soup or, if that is not possible, a slice of melon.

Early Evening

A helping of your special savoury rice.

Dinner

Carbohydrate Meal (serves two)

2 large potatoes for baking
50 g/2 oz parsnips, thinly sliced
50 g/2 oz peas
1 teaspoon sesame oil
2 tablespoons stock

Bake the potatoes in the oven at gas mark 6/200°C/400°F for 1–1¼ hours. When they are ready, stir-fry the parsnips and peas in the oil, then add the stock and cook until absorbed. Cut the potatoes open and spoon in the filling.

Alternative Dinner

Turkey Florentine (serves two)

700 g/1½ lb leaf spinach, chopped, cooked and seasoned with nutmeg, black pepper and 1 clove garlic
6 tomatoes, sliced
2 175 g/6 oz turkey breast fillets

Spread the spinach in the bottom of an ovenproof dish. Arrange the sliced tomato over the spinach and place the turkey breasts on top. Cover and bake at gas mark 5/190°C/375°F for 30 minutes.

Tip of the Day

You may have heard people say, 'Don't eat protein with carbohydrate' and wondered what they meant. Well, there is something in it and it's to do with carbohydrate cravings. If you are the kind of person who gets the occasional urge to binge on sweets, buns, cakes and all sugary things, you are probably a carbohydrate craver. In Part II I will explain the scientific theory behind the term but for here it is enough to say that, when you are trying to satisfy this type of craving you will get better results if you don't mix lots of protein with your (unprocessed) carbohydrate. Follow that advice and you will probably feel better more quickly and the craving will end.

Exercise of the Day

These exercises are for your back, upper arms and particularly your pectoral muscles òn the front of your chest. For women, they may help to raise the bust slightly as well. This is what you do: reach up your back as far as you can with one hand and meet it with the other coming over your shoulder. Now stretch down and try to clasp your hands together. Feel it really stretching your chest and shoulders. Don't worry if you can't make your fingers meet at first, keep trying and, as you loosen up, it will become easier whilst all the time you are exercising your upper body. Try doing it five times a day, three or four times a week to begin with.

Another upper body exercise is slightly easier. Put the palms of your hands together behind your back with the fingers pointing upwards. Start off gradually and see how far you can get up your back. Don't do too much at first; if it hurts stop. Do this one ten times a day.

Treat of the Day

For her: try out various ways to remove hair from your legs – do your own survey and choose the method you like best.

For him: why not treat yourself to a trip to the cinema or theatre, or buy yourself a new CD or album?

Day 7

Breakfast

A bowl of porridge with one slice of melon chopped and sliced into it.

Mid-morning

One plain oat biscuit or one basic biscuit.

Lunch

Spiced Liver Stir-Fry

65 g/2½ oz lambs' or calves' liver cut into strips and marinated for 2 hours

Marinade
1 tablespoon raspberry or wine vinegar
1 tablespoon grapeseed oil
1 teaspoon ground cumin
½ teaspoon ground coriander
Tabasco to taste

Stir fry
2 teaspoons sesame oil
50 g/2 oz carrots
50 g/2 oz bean sprouts
50 g/2 oz courgettes
50 g/2 oz French beans
2 tablespoons chicken stock

Heat the oil and stir-fry the vegetables over a high heat. Add the drained liver for the last 3 or 4 minutes of cooking time.

Alternative Lunch

Rice and lentil salad

125 g/4 oz rice
125 g/4 oz brown or green lentils
4 tomatoes, peeled and chopped
1 bunch spring onions, chopped
1 small bunch coriander, washed and chopped
150 g/5 oz yoghurt
½ lemon, juice only
pepper

Cook the rice and lentils separately. Drain, mix together and allow to cool. Stir in the tomatoes, spring onions, coriander and the yoghurt mixed with the lemon juice. Season with pepper and serve.

If fresh coriander is unavailable, use a dessert-spoon of coriander seeds instead. Roast them in a hot, dry frying pan and crush them with a pestle and mortar. The taste will be different, but just as delicious.

Mid-afternoon

Crunch on a medium-sized apple.

Early Evening

One helping of dahl.

Dinner

Poached Salmon Cutlets (serves two)

2 150 g/5 oz salmon cutlets

Court bouillon
600 ml/1 pint water
1 carrot
1 onion
1 stick celery

1 teaspoon wine vinegar or lemon juice
handful parsley
6 peppercorns

Combine all the ingredients for the court bouillon and heat gently. Cover the cutlets in the warm court bouillon and bring to a simmer – definitely not a boil. Once the liquor is visibly swirling, leave to cook and test with a knife after about 5 minutes. Serve with a cucumber salad made by mixing together ½ cucumber, diced, 150 ml/¼ pint very low-fat natural yoghurt, 1 clove garlic, crushed, 2 teaspoons chopped mint and black pepper.

Alternative Dinner

Grilled Trout (serves two)

2 175 g/6 oz rainbow trout
1 teaspoon grapeseed oil

Stir-fry
2 teaspoons sesame oil
225 g/8 oz fennel, sliced
225 g/8 oz mangetout
225 g/8 oz courgettes
2 tablespoons stock
black pepper

Brush the trout lightly with oil. Heat the grill to high and cook the trout for 7 minutes, turning once. Serve with the vegetable stir-fry.

Tip of the Day

If you really enjoy the taste of salt and are missing it, there's no need to! You can release the natural sodium from a host of fragrant herbs simply by sweating them gently over a low heat with a finely chopped onion. Don't be afraid to use large quantities of fresh herbs in your cooking! For a real taste explosion try chopping some fresh green or red chillis into salads or any dish, but take out the seeds first and be careful to wash your hands before touching your eyes.

Exercise of the Day

There are two exercises today, aimed at helping your back, hips and bottom. For the first one, kneel on the floor, put one hand down and lift the other up in the air at the same time raising your opposite leg. Stretch both arm and leg out straight and hold to the count of five. Then slowly lower them and repeat for the other arm and leg. Do each combination five times.

Next, lie down on your back with your knees in the air and your hands by your side. Now lift your buttocks off the floor as high as you can. Keep them firmly clenched, count to five and slowly lower. Repeat five times. This exercise really does concentrate on the bottom and if you do it every day you will soon get into trim.

Treat of the Day

For her: throw caution to the wind with a totally new lipstick – be daring, get a bright or dark colour you haven't tried before.

For him: how about buying yourself some small weights so you can practise improving those arm muscles?

How to be
Slim and Healthy
for the Rest
of Your Life

Introduction

The weakness in many diets is that they fail to help you maintain your desired weight once you have reached it. Most of us have at some time or other dieted sufficiently strictly to get down to the weight we were aiming for, but nearly everyone will confess that they didn't stay at their ideal weight for long. This is because most diets do not train you to eat in a way which can be sustained happily in the long term. My eating plan is different; while the seven-day diet is fairly rigid, the essential aspects of it still provide an excellent way to continue to eat for the rest of your life. You have already learned about the bonuses of eating this way; you do not feel hungry, you do not get cravings, you do not binge, so, in the long run, you will not put the weight back on. The principles of the seven-day eating plan are so sound that they can be applied to general everyday living, not just to keep you trim but also to keep you in good health.

One of the reasons why people find it difficult sticking to healthy eating is that they believe they have to abandon all their favourite foods for the rest of their lives; this is not true with my eating plan. It is a lifestyle not a life sentence and it is an eating plan not a diet. I have a rule I call the 80/20 rule, passed on to me by an American colleague who is an expert in long-term healthy eating:

IF YOU EAT THE RIGHT FOODS FOR 80 PER CENT OF THE TIME, IT HARDLY MATTERS WHAT YOU EAT FOR THE OTHER 20 PER CENT.

So there is no need to pine for treat foods – you can always have them – and there is no need to deprive yourself to the point where you are overcome by cravings and so binge on them. Remember this rule and it will help you to keep a balanced perspective on what you eat and the way you eat it.

The Eating Plan

Food is not simply the stuff we eat. Our choice of what, where, when and how we eat is shaped by many factors, not all of them within our control. Eating may be one of our most basic body functions but, because of that, it has also evolved into one of the most elaborate rituals of every human culture. Religion, fashion and social convention all play their part in feeding.

Changing our eating habits can be an inconvenience that cuts right through our daily lives and that is one major reason why so many people find ordinary dieting hard work. But with this eating plan it won't be hard work, it will be less painful than you ever imagined. A change to healthier eating habits *on a permanent basis* can be a change to a slimmer, fitter and longer life, not to mention the added bonus of more self-confidence and an improved self-image. For the first time ever you may feel in control of an important part of your life.

This is a guide to healthy eating for everyone, young and old, singles and families, and it is never too late to start. You will feel and see the benefits immediately. I have drawn up easy eating guidelines for you to follow, if you want to, for the rest of your life. *The decision rests with you and you alone.* If you are on a special diet for medical reasons (e.g. diabetes, hypertension, food allergy) or receiving any medication it would be wise to consult your doctor before starting my plan.

But, unless you are in doubt, there's no need to worry because my guidelines are the culmination of years of research, discussions, committees and reports from the experts, interpreted on your behalf. They're also shaped by common sense because, having been a failed dieter all my life, I know the pitfalls and have tried to devise an eating plan based on good science and how the body works but which is nonetheless easy to adhere to.

Because a change in your eating pattern is not something you or your family can do casually, without much thought, it helps to understand the argument in favour of change and the background to what is, essentially, a quiet revolution in dietary wisdom.

To my mind *anything* is easily put into practice if you understand the rationale for it and know why you should follow the rules. I'll be giving you those explanations but first let me deal with a few points on which you may need reassurance.

You've started to lose weight on the first part of

the eating plan (and can continue to trim your body by simply repeating the first seven days) but if you're anything like me, you must be wondering how you're going to keep if off. I honestly don't think I'm exaggerating when I say it isn't going to be difficult, at least not as difficult as you may think and certainly not as difficult as it has been before. I'll even go so far as saying that you won't have to stay on a totally regimented eating plan either. Sounds far fetched? Let me explain.

Why My Eating Plan Will Work in the Long Term

The mainstay of my eating plan is to eat *often and regularly*. There are at least two pay-offs to that: first, you're hardly ever hungry if you eat every two hours and second, as eating gingers up the metabolism of your whole body, you burn up more calories every day than you do when you eat infrequently, and a tremendous amount more than you would if you tried to lose weight by crash diets, starvation diets or microdiets. *Remember, you'll put on weight if you starve; the key to losing weight is EATING.* (See Part I, page 10.) Not eating wholesale, of course, I'm not giving you carte blanche. I mean eating right, in terms of quality and quantity. But you can eat great food, cook delicious recipes, look good and feel good without the usual boring slog.

Changing a Few Bad Habits

You're going to have to change a few habits, of course, but as I describe them you'll know in your heart of hearts they're not a grind.

In fact, I would mistrust anyone who says they're too difficult. Why? Because I tried them on my family (Tom and four sons) and they worked almost without them noticing. Ten years ago, I had just returned from California bursting with enthusiasm for a new heart-healthy diet. At breakfast I announced the new regime saying that at the end of a fortnight's trial we would vote on it. When the two weeks were up I offered, 'Well, how's the skimmed milk going down, the lack of butter, the wholemeal bread ... ?' The responses came, 'What bread?' 'Isn't the milk the same?' 'Didn't miss eggs.' Healthy eating had become the norm, painlessly, for the whole family.

The experience with my own family made me realise that good eating habits which some people dread, for instance no more salt or sugar in or on your food, are much easier to incorporate into your life than you think. There's no need for your food to be less tasty if you take advantage of the natural sodium which is found in all herbs and spices. All you have to do is release that sodium by 'sweating' your herbs, chopped onions, garlic in a dry frying pan and add that mixture to your cooking. Countless people give up sugar in tea and coffee, so why not give it up altogether? In my own case, I gave up sugar seventeen years ago when I first became pregnant. I calculated that I'd eat and drink three-quarters of a ton of sugar in nine months and so I decided that I, and my baby, could well do without that. Use artificial sweeteners if you like.

Dispelling a Few Myths About Food

A new perspective on a few food myths won't do you any harm either. It's crazy to think that lemon juice, grapefruit, pineapple or melon, or any other food for that matter, is itself slimming. That label has stuck either because it was a passing fad based on woolly, unscientific thinking or because it helped to sell a diet. Water retention is thought to be at the root of weight gain but the rule of thumb for you and me is that it never is. It is also thought that initial weight loss is mainly due to water loss. It is if you starve, but it isn't on my eating plan: the weight loss is real, not just water. I recommend you drink lots of water (at least two pints every day) to help you lose weight, in order to keep your kidneys well flushed out so that they can get rid of waste efficiently. Eating as little salt as possible also helps as, for every molecule of salt in the body a molecule of water is retained, and so by cutting down on salt you keep your body water down.

The food you eat can help the body to function well. There are some natural diuretics which pump out water e.g. asparagus, capsicums, parsley, coffee, so include them in your diet. The gummy part of porridge oats (soluble fibre) helps lower your blood cholesterol but so does beetroot, for the same reason. Onions and garlic promote a healthy heart so add them to your cooking. Some foods, like sugar, are totally unnecessary, harmful and give us empty calories with absolutely no nutrition, so why include them?

Carbohydrates – The Foods You Must Eat to Stay Slim

Contrary to most other long-term eating plans mine concentrates on *carbohydrates* (starch), not empty refined starch like white bread, cakes, sweets and so on, but unrefined fresh starches: all fruit and vegetables; wholemeal grains; beans, peas and pulses; brown rice and particularly potatoes. On my eating plan for the rest of your life you can eat the foods that most diets reject. If you want, you can have a carbohydrate blow-out and eat a pound of potatoes.

For very good reasons: it's only following good nutritional theory to make carbohydrates the linchpin of any eating plan: they are bulky and make you feel full; they improve the function of the bowels; they flatten off sudden peaks of high blood sugar which inevitably end in over-compensation with a low blood sugar and a craving. The truth is that the only way to treat a carbohydrate craving is to eat carbohydrate. But not a chocolate bar.

Give your body a bit of time. Be gentle with yourself. Instead eat a potato in its jacket, or a cupful of rice or a plate of dahl. They really do work but you'll have to be mature enough to forego that instant gratification which is a mark of our times.

Carbohydrates are the dieter's best friend because they make you feel good. Proteins don't, which is why it's very difficult to stick to a high protein diet. If you base your eating on carbohydrates as my eating plan suggests you reduce the chances of getting depressed, giving in to a craving, or jacking the whole thing in. So you've got to get carbohydrates (the right ones) into your life. They make controlled eating easier. They give you control. Isn't that an offer too good to refuse? The best way to stay slim is to eat carbohydrates every two hours, for the simple reason that it's working *with* your body instead of *against* it, as most diets do.

The Carbohydrate Story (and Why Carbohydrates Mean 'Happiness' to a Dieter)

* Many foods contain amino-acids, the essential building-blocks of body protein and everyone needs them.
* Carbohydrates contain an amino-acid called tryptophan.
* Tryptophan is needed by the brain to manufacture a chemical called serotonin which lifts

our mood, i.e. carbohydrates tend to make us feel happy. That's why we binge on them if we deprive ourselves of them.

* BUT some of the amino-acids in protein, particularly tyrosine, inhibit the absorption of tryptophan into the brain.
* Hence less serotonin is manufactured in the brain, resulting in a lowering of the mood – i.e. proteins tend to make us less happy, which is why high-protein diets are so difficult to stick to.
* Therefore, keep tryptophan levels up by eating carbohydrate often and protein less often and in small quantities. Also, have protein-free meals.

You will see by now that all the rules of my eating plan have a unifying logic based on sound physiology, which is why it works. (For more details on carbohydrates and mood see pages 152–6.)

Official Nutrition Guidelines

The Long-Term Dietary Goals For All Of Us

The NACNE (National Advisory Committee on Nutrition Education) recommendations, ponderously formulated in 1981 and finally published in 1983, were in the form of long- and short-term goals for the population as a whole and do not specifically cover the needs of any particular person. Children, pregnant women, the elderly and the sick may all need additional advice. The essential message of the report was: do more exercise, cut down on fats, sugars, alcohol and salt, and increase dietary fibre. My long-term eating plan incorporates all that advice so that you may be assured that not only will you be eating to stay trim but you'll be eating healthily as well. What follows is a very brief summary of the long-term goals.

Overweight

* People who exceed the acceptable weight range for their height are jeopardising their health even if they are only mildly overweight.
* All overweight individuals should be more active and take exercise.
* A reduction in food intake is of less value in a programme than a long-term change in the types of foods eaten.

Fat

* Overall, fat consumption should be reduced by about a quarter.
* Consumption of saturated fat should be cut more drastically, in fact nearly halved, from 18 per cent to 10 per cent.
* Consumption of polyunsaturated fat will automatically increase as it is used as a substitute for saturated fats.

Sugar

* Consumption of all sucrose (common brown or white sugar) should also be approximately halved (from 38 kg per annum to 20 kg per annum).
* Sucrose in sweets and snacks should not come to more than half of this new figure.

Fibre

* Adult consumption of fibre should be increased by a half at least.
* Fibre should be taken in the form of wholefoods, cereals, fruit and vegetables rather than simply added as bran.

Salt

* The daily intake of salt should be reduced by ONE THIRD (3–5 g) from the current average level of 8–12 g.

Alcohol

* Consumption should be cut by a third from 6 per cent to 4 per cent of total energy intake, but how can any of us know what this means in real terms? New research indicates that the maximum daily intake should be the equivalent of two glasses of wine for women and double that for men, though rations can be lumped together on occasion.

In addition to these guidelines, I should like to add a few more of my own:

* Never drink alcohol on an empty stomach – even a glass of water will do.

* Avoid high calorie mixers otherwise the tonic will contain more calories than the gin you have it with.
* Always drink an equal quantity of water.
* To avoid a hangover, drink at least a pint of water before sleeping and more if you wake in the night.

Your Personal Eating Plan for the Rest of Your Life

The most up-to-date recommendations we've got, long- and short-term, were not designed for individuals like you and me. What we have to do is adapt them for ourselves and I've tried to do that with some personal guidelines to make changes easy.

When you decide to follow them, your personal goals are up to you as is the length of time over which you make the changes to your diet. Some of the advice is not new. For instance, if you hardly use any sugar already then meeting the goal for sugar may not be too hard and, what's more, there is every reason to cut out sugar completely if you think it's a realistic target.

My own personal recommendations are those that work for me and my family. I can only offer them as that. You will of course have to find your own targets, taking account of your own lifestyle, eating habits and preferences. But, if you look closely at my guidelines, I hope you will see how you can apply the general goals to a set of personal objectives you can easily live with.

My Basic Guidelines for a Slimmer, Fitter, Healthier Life

* Eat more fresh fruit, vegetables and fish and less processed food.
* Eat six times a day. Make each meal a ritual. Sit down at the table, make a place setting, invite a friend to make it a social occasion.
* Take your food seriously, give it the benefit of your full attention, especially at meals. Don't watch television or read a newspaper. Chew food thoroughly.
* Make breakfast a good meal by eating cereal either hot or cold e.g. porridge or a sugar-free brand of muesli or flakes. Oats are particularly good for you with their soluble fibre.
* Eat more beans and pulses instead of fatty red meat or full-fat cheese. Plant protein is as good as animal protein! It isn't 'second-class', as outdated theories suggested.
* Use smaller portions of red meat and fatty cheeses as a condiment to accompany green

and root vegetables and rice or wholemeal pasta and boiled potatoes.

* At any meal, eat vegetables first and drink two glasses of water.
* Eat more wholegrain products and less processed and refined foods (especially junk food).
* Try healthy foreign foods e.g. Greek, Japanese, genuine Indian.
* Give up sugar and salt, remove them from the dining table and stop using them in cooking.
* If you buy them at all, be aware of the hidden sugar and salt in processed foods. Read food labels carefully and don't buy products which have added sugar or salt.
* To keep your heart and lungs in good shape, your muscles toned up and your stamina reliable, take moderate exercise for at least twenty minutes and preferably thirty minutes, four times a week. Remember, this has the added pay-off of keeping your metabolism up so that you burn more calories all the time – even when you're asleep.
* If you get a craving for something sweet, try sating it with some unprocessed carbohydrate, either fruit, raw vegetables (e.g. carrots) or some cooked 'bulk food' like rice or dahl. Wait for half an hour after eating a little and you'll find your craving has gone (see page 62 in Part I).

Treat Sweets

For the incorrigible sweet tooth, here are a couple of recipes for sweet treats which can be consumed once or twice a week instead of sweets, chocolate, ice cream etc. One could be eaten during the seven-day diet if in extremis!

Apricot and Orange Balls (makes about 24)

450 g/1 lb dried apricots, chopped
1 medium orange, peeled and chopped
65 g/2½ oz grated coconut
65 g/2½ oz ground nuts

Mix all the ingredients together – if possible, mince them in a food processor. Shape the mixture into 24 small balls. Chill until firm.

Chewy Fruit

400 g/14 oz dried apricots, soaked, or fresh fruit,
 peeled and cored or 800 g/28 oz tinned fruit in
 natural juices

Preheat the oven to its lowest setting. Purée the
fruit and then cook it over a low heat for 5 minutes.
Cover a baking tray with cling film and put the fruit
in the centre. Spread evenly across the tray. Bake
in the oven for about 8 hours until the fruit
becomes dry and chewy. Peel off the cling film and
cut into shapes. Store in the refrigerator.

Eight Tips on How to Cheat Your Appetite

* Eat before you get hungry.
* Always serve your food on a small plate.
* Eat vegetables/salad/fruit first, meat later.
* Eat very slowly to allow the carbohydrates to act and turn off your appetite.
* If you want to nibble, eat rice, pulses or cold potatoes.
* Drink water all through the day and especially through meals.
* Drink still water rather than fizzy water.
* Put oats, kidney beans and beetroot on the menu, and anything else that contains lots of soluble fibre.

Some Difficult Meals and How to Cope With Them

Ah, that's all very well, you're saying, but life isn't always like that. What about the business lunch? What about not having time for anything but a snack, eating on the run? Do I resort to old bad habits? You needn't. Here's how.

The Business Lunch

The key to the successful business lunch is to see it as a treat to have the most delicious food, which is also healthy and low in calories:

Aperitif

* Large glass of mineral water, which starts to fill you up.

Starters

* Smoked salmon.
* Gravad lax.
* Half an Ogen melon.
* Gorgeous salads (ask for dressing on the side so that you can add only what you want).
* Fresh prawns.

Main Course

* Always fish but choose the nicest (e.g. monkfish, turbot, halibut, swordfish).
* At least *four* vegetables (exclude potatoes this time). They help to satisfy you so eat them FIRST.
* No fancy sauces.
* Any amount of fancy salad.

Pudding

* Always fresh fruit but choose the most appetising and exotic e.g. mango, papaya, passion fruit, guavas, raspberries and strawberries out of season.

Wine

* 1 glass white } not every day of course
* 1 glass red

Water

* Drink at least equal quantities of water as wine, plus one glass.

Coffee

* No cream.

Digestives

* Pass on the port and brandy.

Food on the Run

* In your bag keep an apple, banana and/or a small piece of Edam cheese.
* Stop at the greengrocers for half a pound of your favourite fruit and eat on the run.
* Ask sandwich bars to use:
    * wholemeal bread
    * no butter or marge
    * no dressing of any kind
    * lots of black pepper.
* Drop into the Greek place and grab a pitta with a little meat and lots of salad.
* Drop into the Indian for a dish of dahl.
* Ask the Chinese for a dish of mixed vegetables or even some rice on its own.
* Eat a low-calorie diabetic bar.
* Drink half a pint of skimmed milk.

* Have a pot of flavoured very low-calorie yoghurt plus a plain wholemeal bun or bap.
* Have a pot of any salad, but leave as much of the dressing as you can. Don't be content with the standard canteen salad of a lettuce leaf, half a tomato and a piece of egg.

Exercise in Your Life

Eating sensibly is 50 per cent of being trim for the rest of your life but it isn't everything. Almost as important is exercise – and that's easy too if you just look for opportunities to incorporate it into your lifestyle, some of which I've already mentioned in Part I.

* Never use a lift or escalator again.
* Walk, then run, then leap two at a time up stairs.
* Stride out whenever you can.
* Always do your tummy and pelvic floor exercises (see pages 63 and 69).
* Get some active sport going. One that you like such as tennis, squash, badminton, netball, skiing or offer to be the referee at the local sports club.
* Find some exercise to do at home (exercise bicycle, rowing machine) that you really like to do and do it for twenty to thirty minutes, four times a week.

Making the Change to Healthier Eating

The benefits of a healthy lifestyle based on regular exercise and a good diet will quickly become apparent and, like me, you'll probably wonder how you ever managed to get by previously. You will feel better and find you have more energy. But switching to a healthy lifestyle will put you in the vanguard of the nation's health movement and by becoming a forward thinker you will have to put up with other more backward thinkers all around you. In practice this means that you have to rely more on yourself and less on others for your healthy diet.

However, all of us have nagging doubts about how feasible the changes are. How much hardship is involved? Will the inconvenience be too much? Will restrictions be demoralising? Well, there have been a number of studies looking at how well people cope with changing to healthy eating. One which I found particularly interesting involved a group of nearly 500 dieticians and their families, who, instead of changing gradually, agreed to make the switch overnight.

Of course, some found it easier than others, to make the changes. Many thought they could adjust to the new eating pattern for the rest of their lives. Many remarked on the need to eat larger meals more frequently because the food they were now eating was not as rich in calories as their previous diet. That is what happens when you substitute unprocessed carbohydrates such as root vegetables, wholegrains, rice, pulses and beans for rich fatty foods and refined sugary foods.

It's good news for anybody who is overweight because eating the right foods automatically reduces your calorie intake – even if you feel you are eating more volume overall. What's more, although there are fewer calories, there are more nutrients so you win both ways!

Every change works best if you're prepared. We found that when I made a TV series on how to give up smoking. So I feel I must warn you about your hardest task. Substituting unprocessed starchy food for rich, fatty foods is the single most important aspect of the transition to healthier eating and, as the dieticians' study revealed, this is the switch that also takes the most effort. After all, the message to cut down on sugar, in the name of less dental decay, has only been really successful in the last few years. Given that saturated fat has been exposed as a 'villain' comparatively recently and the mistaken victim, starch, has been allowed a slow rehabilitation, it's going to take a little time for that message to build in strength and be acted on.

Quite apart from the mental adjustment needed when planning menus along the new guidelines, the dieticians found that they had to be careful about shopping and had to stockpile healthy snacks whenever they came across them as not all food stores stock them. Forewarned is to be forearmed!

I suggest that you set yourself a timetable for the transition. Don't try to do everything at once – if you intend to convert your family with you, you will certainly have to take care to take things gradually.

How to Put Your New Eating Plan into Action

Fat

* Start by cutting down on fatty meals: grill food rather than fry, eat more baked potatoes and fewer chips, start using skimmed milk instead of full-cream milk if you haven't already.
* Make sure that the oil you use is polyunsaturated (e.g. sunflower, maize or soya oil) and not just labelled 'vegetable oil', since that may be a blend containing saturated oil.
* Use a polyunsaturated margarine and spread it thinly over wholemeal bread.

None of these changes will be news to you but they will help adjust the mix of fat to starch.

Meat

* Stop cooking 'meat and two veg' meals. Start cooking more vegetables with less meat.
* Go for more white meat and fish or leaner cuts of the red meats.
* But be careful: even 'lean' beef, pork and lamb contain high percentages of fat. Sausages, mince, burgers and pâtés are very high in fat, much of it saturated.
* Liver, kidneys and offal in general tend to be far less fatty than red meat, so eat more of these.
* When you cook chicken or other fowl, don't eat the skin, which is rich in fat.
* Stir-fries are an excellent way to make a tasty meal using less meat and less fat. You only need a little oil and seasoning in a hot wok. Stir-frying is also more economical on heat and makes washing-up simpler.

Salt

* Phase out salt over a fortnight.
* If you really must have salt, use much less and use it only while cooking.
* Never leave chopped vegetables to stand in salted water and throw away salted vegetable water.
* Beans, pulses and lentils will cook more quickly and without hardening if you cut out salt.

* If you cook pasta in salted water, rinse it with boiling water before serving.
* If food tastes flat to begin with, be patient. Give your palate time to reset at a new level. Once you and your family have adjusted to low-salt or salt-free cooking, you'll wonder what all the fuss was about.
* And don't just leave it at that, experiment! There are many ways to enhance and supplement the natural flavours of food without resorting to salt. Herbs and spices are particularly good and there are so many to choose from. Try using black pepper, paprika, nutmeg, cumin or a mixture of spices.
* Of course, there are low-sodium salts (based on potassium instead of sodium) which can help some people but I hesitate to recommend them for non-medical diets since it seems to me to be an admission of defeat.
* Banishing the salt-cellar from the house is not the end of the matter. Most of the salt we eat is already included in food produce: bacon and smoked fish and meats are quite high in salt; pickles, sauces, ready-made soups and most of the savoury snack foods like nuts, crisps and nibbles are all quite heavily salted. So cut down on these processed foods.
* Be careful: other sources of salt are less obvious. Tinned fish and vegetables, breakfast cereals and the harder cheeses can also contain appreciable quantities of salt.
* Remember, we are not trying to remove *all* salt

from the diet – a little salt is an absolute physiological necessity. However, you are unlikely to suffer from a salt deficiency in twentieth-century Britain.

Sugar

* Sucrose is without any nutritional value whatsoever.
* White and brown sugar (sucrose) are foods to be avoided completely.
* But it's not quite as simple as that: even if you throw away the sugar bowl, there is still quite a lot left to do. Sugar alone or when added to processed food comes in many forms other than that labelled 'sucrose'. These other forms, which are all just as much of a problem as sucrose, include glucose, maltose, fructose, any syrup (e.g. dextrose, glucose), and any form of sugar whether or not it is called unrefined e.g. cane sugar, molasses, muscovado, demerara. These sugars permeate a huge proportion of the food industry's products as their ability to enhance flavours is highly prized. It's important that you become aware of quite how extensively sugar is used.
* About 60 per cent of the hundreds of millions of tons of sugar consumed in the UK each year is eaten in the form of processed foods. Of course, chocolate and all sweets account for a large part of that consumption; a large propor-

tion of the rest comes from biscuits, sweet pastries, cakes, jams and other spreads, pickles, chutneys, sauces.

* Most bottled drinks have a high sugar content, as do most puddings and dessert dishes.
* Unless natural yoghurt is specifically labelled 'very low fat' it is very likely to have added sugar.
* Most of the popular processed breakfast cereals have a surprisingly high sugar content. A few make a point of being sugar-free – look out for them.
* Because sugar is such an excellent preservative, many tinned foods are canned in syrup, so beware!

Decision Time – It's Up To You

There is little point in giving you a long list of 'don't's' and, anyway, I don't believe I should proscribe your food. The only way to lose weight and stay slim is to control your intake of energy-rich foods, namely fats and sugars. If you adopt my guidelines I know you'll find the food both appetising and filling and, even more importantly, you'll find it's much easier than you imagined to take control of your eating pattern.

Look at your present eating habits and decide where you can make appropriate substitutions. Remember, though, even as you eat more and more fresh fruit and vegetables as your primary source of sugar, whenever you do eat a sugary snack you are adding calories with little or no nutritional value.

Slowly the food industry is responding to the growing demand for low-sugar or sugar-free products. Many tinned fruits are now available in fruit juice, still rich in natural sugar but a great improvement on syrup. Sugar-free baked beans are also now widely available and make an excellent convenience food. It's up to you to check what you are buying. Look at the labels and if it's not clear, ask the manager. It's only by customers bringing the issue to their attention that the retailers will increase their range of low-sugar or sugar-free products.

I know that cutting down on sugar may be the hardest change for you to make. Please persevere! Sugar is such a potent food that the body does acquire a sugar habit and it will take time to readjust. What's more, the mechanism for this habit is now becoming fairly well understood and if you read page 151 you will see how altering your sugar intake can not only help you lose weight or keep slim but also help you avoid headaches and much else. And remember, my 80/20 rule (see page 92) will allow you to indulge occasionally.

The Changing Patterns of
Diet and Disease

Several million years ago, when our ancestors were scratching out a living in the African plains, their diet consisted largely of fruit, nuts and other vegetables. Whether as hunters or scavengers, they ate little meat and were, in the main, gatherers. Our teeth testify to their omnivorous eating habits and so, less obviously, does our digestive system.

It was a menu of fresh fruit and vegetables as available, topped up with the occasional blow-out of meat. Unlike us they probably spent a good deal of their time munching because vegetation is not a rich source of calories.

Now the world is a much more crowded place. In the United Kingdom, hunger is no longer such a widespread problem: quite the opposite. Today, the Western world has replaced malnutrition through insufficiency with malnutrition and disease through excess.

Obesity first became noticeable among the upper classes in the nineteenth century but the most dramatic transition in our national eating habits came after the Second World War. The post-war boom in agriculture saw a massive increase in the production and consumption of meat and dairy products. Ironically, the period of food rationing had produced a diet that was remarkably beneficial but all the benefit vanished as people gratefully switched away from bulky vegetable meals to more energy-rich and fatty foods.

Now we have, at least in Scotland, reasonable claim to the title of Heart Attack Blackspot of the World. The incidence of coronary heart disease, obesity, hypertension, diabetes and all the other 'diseases of affluence and over-eating' (diverticular disease, constipation, piles, cancer of the colon, gallstones, to name a few in the digestive system) has risen in the UK in direct correlation with our change to a more refined, energy-rich, fatty diet.

How can we be sure that our diet is to blame for these twentieth-century deathstyles? After all, hardly anything has remained the same in our lives since the war. Evidence gathered from the study of other people's eating habits and patterns of disease can be quite persuasive. Certainly, although we are all one species, these patterns of diet and disease vary dramatically from one culture to another.

The traditional diet of one of the last remaining

hunters, the Eskimo, consists largely of meat, agriculture being rather difficult in the ice-floes. Yet, despite a lifetime of meat and blubber, the incidence of heart attacks is very low. The difference may well be due to the source of the meat: fish not animal meat. In rural Africa and South America, heart disease is also rare but, as Westernisation proceeds, so the incidence increases. The same has happened in Japan. Twenty-five years ago the Japanese diet of mainly fish and vegetables kept the nation virtually heart attack-free. But in a quarter of a century we've seen the effect of switching to a Western diet – the incidence of heart attacks is approaching that in the West.

Perhaps the most compelling evidence comes from comparing ourselves with other developed countries. Finland used to have the highest death rate from coronary heart disease until they changed their eating habits as a nation. Similarly, across Western Europe and the USA, people have adjusted their diet and the incidence of heart disease has dropped. So why have we in Britain been so slow to change our eating habits? To a degree, we've been led astray by bad advice, especially in the vexed area of heart-healthy eating.

The Heart-healthy Diet

There can be few people today who doubt that what they eat can affect their health. In the light of this, the marked reluctance of many experts to commit themselves to clear, unequivocal guidance on what foods should be avoided and what foods should be sought is appalling. Unfortunately, the last place to look for guidance is the Department of Health and many in the medical profession have also signally failed to demystify an area of long-standing and unnecessary confusion.

Our choice of food, the way we choose to cook it and, especially, the amount we eat does indeed affect our health. The wrong eating pattern combined with other bad habits such as smoking, drinking to excess and insufficient exercise, can lead to disease and early death. The most striking correlation between what we eat and illness is between saturated fat (found almost entirely in meat and dairy products) and coronary heart disease. The connection is made through that infamous and much maligned intermediate, cholesterol.

Cholesterol lies at the centre of the great diet/disease debate. Speaking in general terms, the more saturated fat you eat, the more cholesterol will be found in your bloodstream; the higher the (serum) cholesterol level, the greater the risk of an early death from coronary heart disease – even though it is only one of several risk factors and our cholesterol level is mainly determined by cholesterol manufactured inside the body.

In coronary heart disease the build-up of fat in the lining of the coronary arteries (atheroma) gradually reduces their internal bore and consequently the blood supply to the muscles of the heart itself. Some people experience severe chest pains (angina) in the weeks preceding a heart attack; others get no early warning. The heart attack happens when one of the major coronary arteries is completely blocked by a blood clot (thrombus) forming (in a matter of hours) around a particularly prominent fatty deposit (atheromatous plaque) on the lining of the artery wall.

The important point is this: there is a wealth of data, accumulated over decades, to support these findings, namely that the level of cholesterol in the bloodstream is our best indicator of the risk of coronary heart disease. This is not the same thing as saying that cholesterol causes heart attacks. Few scientists are satisfied that cause and effect has been proven. Even if it is entirely free of blame, however, cholesterol, as an indicator, tells us to cut down on our dietary intake of fats – particularly saturated fats – because that will reduce our risk of heart disease, and that is the simple and vital take-home message.

As I have said before, Britain has one of the worst death rates from coronary heart disease in the world. It is the number one cause of death in the UK. In 1987 it accounted for approximately 31 per cent of deaths in men and 24 per cent of deaths in women. The USA also had a very high incidence of coronary heart disease in the seventies but they have already changed their eating habits and have seen considerable change – for the better – in the last fifteen years. Exact comparisons are difficult but while the figures for men in England and Wales have dropped by less than 9 per cent since 1976, in the USA there has been a drop of about 33 per cent.

The UK death rate from coronary heart disease has remained at about the same level because people continue to eat the same food, including the same unacceptably high levels of fats (42 per cent of total energy). But is there any reason to suppose that the British are so peculiarly intransigent, to the point of death, when compared with their peers in Europe and the USA? The truth is that, when it comes to coronary heart disease, Britain has an appalling record of health education. Despite nine major reports on diet and health in the last twelve years there are still no comprehensive practical national dietary goals. The one and only report in forty years to give dietary advice was circulated only amongst professionals.

The net result has been compromise, confusion and inaction, a situation that suited several different interested parties and lobbies and it is hard to believe that there was not an element of wilful obstruction from some participants. This is not to lay the blame solely at the door of the most obvious vested interests represented by the farmers, the food manufacturers and the retail and tobacco industries: even some health educators were not anxious to adopt initiatives to prevent coronary heart disease.

Shopping

Food Labels

If you want to have more control over what you eat you are going to have to look more carefully at what you buy off the shelf in your supermarkets. Have a look at some packets in your freezer and some tins in your cupboards.

At the moment the information on the labels varies widely. The only compulsory information required by law is a list of ingredients and some food additives including flavourings, colourings, preservatives, emulsifiers, stabilisers, thickeners and artificial sweeteners. Not many people realise that the ingredients have to be listed in descending order of weight. Water must be included as an ingredient if it is more than 5 per cent by weight of the food.

Not all foods have to have this information. Whole fresh fruit and vegetables, honey, hen's eggs, coffee and coffee products, vinegar, milk, cheese, butter and fermented dairy products free of extra ingredients are exempted. Less obviously, cocoa and chocolate products and condensed and dried milk products are also exempt.

Nutritional information is still voluntary although more and more manufacturers are offering some as their consumers become more health conscious. Usually nutritional information is limited to a breakdown into calorific value (i.e. the available energy in the product) and then percentage values for total fat, total carbohydrate and protein. Sometimes the manufacturer will state the amount of salt and fibre as well. The voluntary guidelines for declaring nutritional information suggest showing these values for a 100 g portion or by the whole or a fraction of the product (i.e. per can, carton, box).

Unfortunately some of the most useful nutritional information is not available. It is not easy to find separate values for soluble sugars (glucose, dextrose, etc.) as distinct from insoluble and unrefined starch (cellulose, lignin). All are lumped together as carbohydrates. Similarly, outside the butter/margarine and cooking oil battleground, fats are not often broken down into saturated and polyunsaturated.

Even if we do see an improvement in labelling standards, perhaps when we adopt a European standard in or after 1992, it will not be a substitute for your own careful scrutiny. Remember, if a product says 'no added sugar' that doesn't mean it's sugar-free. Adding tomato sauce and fruit juices are two ways of sweetening products and, while they are preferable to the addition of neat sucrose, they are in themselves processed foods stripped free of dietary fibre and rich in calories.

Remember, too, that if a processed food boasts of the minerals and vitamins it has added to it – perhaps a significant proportion of the recommended daily amount – it is probably because they were lost from the food (along with the fibre) in the original processing.

Food Storage

As you eat more and more fresh fruit, vegetables and fish, your shopping habits will probably have to change.

* Make more frequent regular visits to the green-grocer and support your local fishmonger!
* Fish is especially good eaten the day it is caught so don't keep it waiting in the fridge.
* Pulses and beans can be kept in Kilner jars for months but they will lose nutrients and take longer to cook, so buy them in relatively small quantities and replenish your supplies as necessary.
* Stocks and pulse dishes can take some time to cook, so prepare them in batches and keep them in the freezer. If you have a microwave, they can be quickly thawed and reheated.

Nutrition: Fact and Fancy

Energy and nutrition

In order to understand how my eating plan works, you need to know a little bit about the human body, how it uses food and what sort of food it needs. The first thing to get straight is the distinction between food for nutrition and food for energy.

There are certain components of food that the body cannot function without. Vitamin C, for instance, which keeps mucous membranes healthy, and a deficiency of which can lead to scurvy; vitamin B12, a lack of which will cause damage to the nerves; calcium, a lack of which will lead to rickets and osteoporosis; and iron, a lack of which will lead to anaemia. Not surprisingly, these are called the 'essential nutrients' and include the minerals and vitamins you see on some food labels.

Then there is energy. There is no such thing as a

perfectly efficient process and every physical, chemical or biological change that takes place in your body means that you use up energy, which has to be replenished by food.

A standard wallchart used by biochemists shows a summary of the thousands of different, interlinked chain reactions that are going on in the human body all the time. Along each pathway some molecules are built up whilst others are broken down and recycled again. All these reactions make up the 'metabolic processes'. It's carefully colour coded for clarity but it still succeeds in making the map of the London Underground look simple by comparison. Every reaction in the body needs energy to drive it. That's why you need a certain amount of energy every day simply to carry on normal existence whether that involves exercise or not. Different foodstuffs have varying value as sources of nutrition and energy. Some foods, such as fruit and vegetables, are extremely nutritious but fairly low on energy; others, like sugar, are very high in energy and low on nutrition. So it pays to eat a large amount of the former and little of the latter.

As far as the body is concerned there are three major categories of food: fats, proteins and carbohydrates. Because each of these is processed in different ways it has long been convenient to talk of food in these biochemical terms. Unfortunately, part of the confusion over what constitutes a good diet has been precisely because we have insisted in seeing a food as a source of protein or starch rather than as a source of nutrition with a wide variety of useful and not so useful components. One such food is liver, which is an excellent source of protein, vitamins and minerals but also of undesirable cholesterol.

To take another example, until recently, cheese was recognised as a valuable source of protein. Now, many people recognise it as a potential source of undesirably high levels of saturated fat. Depending on the cheese, either or both of these outlooks may be justified but neither has helped develop an easy understanding of good nutrition. Cheese is a processed dairy product. Like all animal produce, dairy or meat, cheese has enjoyed an unjustifiably high level of prestige as the powerful food lobby of farmers, manufacturers and retailers have promoted their interests.

One unfortunate spin-off of this post-war promotion of cheese, full-cream milk, eggs and meat as staple items of our diet has been the entirely erroneous idea that somehow plant proteins are inferior to animal proteins. All proteins are made of the same component parts, some twenty-two different amino-acids. Neither plants nor animals nor the human digestive system make any distinction between animal- or plant-derived amino-acids. They can't because they are identical.

Protein

Proteins are the building-blocks of the body and are not used as a source of energy unless the body is in a desperate situation (i.e. starving). The body uses amino-acids to construct a vast number of different protein structures. Compared with fats or carbohydrates, there is a much greater diversity of shapes and sizes. Indeed, it's the shape of a protein that determines its principal function. Enzymes, antibodies, the mass of muscle, skin, cartilage, blood and other tissues all comprise protein in large part. Because all the body's proteins are continually broken down into amino-acids and rebuilt in an inefficient way, the body needs a daily regular supplement of protein.

Eight of the twenty-two amino-acids cannot be made in the body from other substrates (the rest can). These eight are called essential amino-acids and a good diet must include them. In general, animal products tend to have a more even spread of the different amino-acids and more of the essential ones, whereas plants may 'major' in particular ones at the expense of others. For instance, cereals tend to be low in lysine, one of the essential amino-acids but happily beans and pulses are rich in lysine. A vegetarian diet must therefore contain a very wide variety of vegetables to provide all the amino-acids; only a little meat will provide the same cover. All in all, in twentieth-century Great Britain, there is not really any problem in meeting the recommended daily amounts of protein, even if you don't eat much meat or cheese.

Despite this, whilst latterday experts enthused about cheese and animal protein, cereals were classed as 'starch' and the notion that they could be an important source of protein was hardly considered. Of course, due to our predilection for highly processed and refined foods such as white flour, there wasn't very much protein left in cereal products anyway.

Times have changed. Everybody knows that wholemeal bread is good for you even if they still prefer to eat anaemic sliced white bread. But the legacy of that unfortunate underestimation of plants as sources of protein is still very much alive and needs to be firmly rebutted. Now that high levels of saturated fats are so strongly implicated in coronary heart disease the tables are turning. That is why any eating plan with its emphasis on unprocessed carbohydrates, fruit, vegetables and pulses, with meat added only as a condiment, is so appropriate if you want to keep your heart healthy.

Fats

Fat provides the body with energy in its most concentrated form. We are all familiar with fat as adipose tissue; many of us are too familiar with it. But, apart from its role as an energy store, the components of fat play a vital part in many of our fundamental metabolic processes.

Fats are made of triplets of fatty acids linked together by a unit of glycerol. The fatty acids can be saturated or unsaturated depending on how 'saturated' they are with hydrogen atoms. Saturated fatty acids tend to be harder and solid at room temperature. Polyunsaturates are thinner and liquid at room temperature. With the exception of coconut and palm oils, almost all plant-derived oils are polyunsaturated or mono-unsaturated.

The principal source of saturated fat is animal produce. At present, the government, through the Common Agricultural Policy, is subsidising the production of food with high levels of saturated fat. The butter mountain, for example, is 65 per cent saturated fat. The milk lake is similar. There are, however, no subsidies to encourage the production of leaner meat as yet. One day, perhaps, the Department of Health will have a word with the Ministry of Agriculture, Fisheries and Food. In the meantime, the only way you the customer can have any effect is by voting with your feet and demanding lean meat from your butcher or only buying the leaner cuts at supermarkets. Better still, leave red meat alone and eat fowl, fish and pulses instead.

Just as some amino-acids cannot be made by the body, so certain fatty acids are essential to the diet. These essential fatty acids are all polyunsaturates. One in particular, linoleic acid, is the precursor for a production line that gives rise to several very important classes of molecules including arachidonic acid found in the membranes of every cell and its downstream product the prostaglandins, a group which regulates myriad vital functions. Everyone's diet should include foods which contain these essential fatty acids, foods such as oily fish, vegetable oils and nuts.

Fats, Cholesterol and Coronary Heart Disease

As we have seen, in recent years there has been increasing concern over the role of saturated fat in the development of coronary heart disease, our single greatest cause of death today. The concern revolves around the different way saturated and unsaturated fats are transported about the body in the bloodstream. Because fats (lipids) are insoluble in water they have to be combined with protein, making a 'lipoprotein', in order to get around the bloodstream. But there is a third component in this transport system: cholesterol. As I mentioned earlier, there has been a great deal of confusion and premature judgement on the culpability of cholesterol in coronary heart disease. Much of this arises from its close association with fat in lipoproteins.

When lipids are travelling to or from adipose tissue (the stores of fat we are all trying to limit) or muscle, they have, relatively speaking, a very low density. These lipoproteins are therefore logically enough called 'very low-density lipoproteins'. After the fatty part has been delivered, its place is taken by cholesterol in the blood and it becomes merely a 'low density lipoprotein'. Finally, the transport system can load up with extra protein for some journeys making 'high density lipoprotein'. Dangerous cholesterol deposits are derived from low density lipoprotein carriers (LDLs). If your LDL level is high, your risk of a heart attack is raised.

It has become clear that for people with very high levels of serum cholesterol, reducing the total amount of fat they eat in their diet, particularly the amount of saturated fat, does help to lower their serum cholesterol level and that does reduce their risk of heart attack. In short, they live longer. This evidence comes simply from long-term studies of groups of high-risk people who either did or did not change their dietary habits.

Most of us have much lower levels of serum cholesterol but levels that none the less constitute a significant risk factor for heart disease. What is not yet established is whether we too can derive the same benefit from a fairly drastic change in diet, namely cutting down on fat generally and substituting saturated fats with polyunsaturated fats.

My own view, however, is that we should go ahead and alter our diets because there are many *other* benefits from a reduction in fats not the least being that you'll cut many calories from your diet, fats being the most calorific foods. Whilst polyunsaturates may not be a complete panacea (they contain just the same amount of calories as saturates) for the time being at least they are certainly healthier. Fish oils are the healthiest as the oil seems to protect against heart disease and I recommend that you eat oily fish twice a week on the plan.

Carbohydrates, Sugar and Fibre

To lessen your confusion, you should know that the following words are used interchangeably, even synonymously, by scientists: carbohydrate equal sugar, starch or cellulose, depending on the context.

Whereas fat is reasonably easy to recognise in food, the whole picture is much murkier when it comes to carbohydrates. All the sugars, starch (potatoes, apples), cellulose (the stringy bits in vegetables like celery), gum, pectin (the gummy component of fruit which makes jam set) and many other compounds are members of the carbohydrate family. Essentially, they are all made from simple sugar units like glucose or its near relatives and they all, ultimately, come from the interaction of the sun with plants courtesy of photosynthesis. Whilst the sugars with small molecules like fructose (fruit sugar) and lactose (milk sugar) are water-soluble, the larger – the polysaccharides like starch and cellulose – are insoluble. Apart from two important secondary sources of sugar – honey and breast milk – we should continue to get all our carbohydrate from fruits and vegetables, in other words plant material.

Plants have cellulose as we have skeletons, to provide them with a framework of support – for instance the 'wood' of trees. They use large-moleculed starch to store energy and they use the small-moleculed soluble sugars to transport energy and release it. The human body can digest sugar and, if it's cooked or fermented, it can digest starch but it *cannot* break down cellulose. Cellulose remains in the gut as 'fibre' or bulk.

From the mid-nineteenth century onwards we tended to regard cellulose and all the other indigestible bits of plants as inconveniences to be avoided. Great store was put on refined and more easily digestible extracts of plants, such as white flour, white rice, peeled potatoes. By refining plant material we isolate the energy sources and concentrate them. The most concentrated and refined source of carbohydrate energy is, of course, sugar.

Until the seventies, this urge to refine foods was thought to be 'a good thing' but now we know better. By separating the essential energy of plants from all the rest, we not only lose all the nutritional components – valuable protein, minerals, vitamins and oils – but we also lose the fibre.

The medical significance of fibre has been known for more than twenty-five years but it came back with a vengeance with Audrey Eyton's *F-Plan* diet, the most successful diet for a long time. Fibre is now recognised to have several valuable properties.

The most obvious is the bulk effect. Bran and the other non-available carbohydrates in plants that go to make up fibre bulk up the contents of our intestines and so make our stools less dense and softer. This can lead to a bloated feeling when you first increase the amount of dietary fibre in your meals but there are many positive benefits which outweigh this temporary discomfort. In the undeveloped world, where unrefined plant material, in the form of roots and wholegrain cereals, make up most of the diet, conditions like diverticular disease, haemorrhoids and appendicitis – even bowel cancers – are virtually unknown because passing stools is not such a strain as it can be with our constipation-prone Western diet.

Dietary fibre also acts as a cleansing agent as it passes through the digestive tract not, as you might guess, like a brush but more like a sponge, absorbing waste as it goes. This is because much of what we regard as roughage is actually soluble and forms a sticky, viscous gel in the gut, a bit like a porridge. In fact the similarity is not a coincidence. Oats are one of the richest sources of soluble fibre (kidney beans and beetroot are others), which is precisely why I include them in my recommended diet.

Whilst it is thought that the sticky mass of fibre moving through the gut can mop up all sorts of toxic and potentially hazardous compounds, it is now well established that a regular diet rich in soluble fibre can also reduce the level of low density lipoproteins in the bloodstream. Quite apart from the implications for the risk of coronary heart disease, a reduction in circulating cholesterol also implies a reduction in the risk of gallstones (formed from crystals of cholesterol).

Another consequence of eating a reasonable amount of fibre is that food passes through the gut more quickly. Thus any unpleasant toxins or potential carcinogens have less time to act on the lining of the gut. This may help us understand the cause of colon and bowel cancer. Cancer of the colon is yet another disease of the affluent countries which shows significant correlation with diet, both with high levels of fat and low levels of dietary fibre. Although we can't yet with absolute certainty isolate a particular culprit, it is a further argument for prudent adjustment of both.

Finally, there is one more extremely important bonus that comes of eating food in a more natural and bulkier form. The goodness within it is surrendered *gradually*. The gut absorbs sugar in the form of glucose. The rate at which your blood glucose level rises after a meal affects your health and your mood, so by eating wholefoods you get fewer troughs of low blood sugar when cravings can arise.

Sugar, Diabetes, Liquid Lunches and Headaches

Glucose is the form in which energy is transported to all tissues. Some of it is stored in the liver and muscles as glycogen for use when the body needs an extra energy boost quickly. Unlike fat, which only yields its energy slowly, glycogen can be quickly broken down into glucose within minutes and acts as our principal short-term energy reserve.

To put it in perspective, fat will get you through a period of famine, and glycogen will help you run a few miles. When the blood is too rich in glucose, the hormone insulin converts the excess to glycogen, or if the glycogen reserves in the liver are complete, the glucose will be converted to fat. When blood glucose levels are too low, the hormone glucagon mobilises the glycogen in the liver to form glucose, which then passes into the blood.

Since the advent of refined sugar our bodies have come to rely much more on the regulating role of insulin. Among the diseases of affluence, adult-onset diabetes is yet another that shows a striking association with our Western diet. The incidence in undeveloped countries is very low but rises markedly with urbanisation and the consumption of more refined foodstuffs. In Britain, there are about half a million registered adult-onset diabetics and the real figure is certainly larger. It may be that the sheer concentration of glucose rapidly absorbed into the bloodstream and assaulting the beta cells of the pancreas (where insulin is synthesised and released) is a direct cause of the disease.

We in the Western world seem to have developed a tolerance – a habit – to much stronger concentrations of blood glucose than the levels to which our bodies have been accustomed through evolution. When levels begin to drop, we may have cravings for sweet foods or anything that serves the same purpose (e.g. alcohol). Short of intravenous injection, swallowing carbohydrate in a soluble form, as sucrose for instance, is the best way to get a 'quick fix' – and this is exactly reflected in the way people talk about needing chocolate or other sweets.

The trouble with getting glucose in such a way is that the massive sudden influx into the bloodstream triggers the release of large quantities of insulin in an attempt to stabilise the level. Two hours or so after your chocolate snack or liquid lunch, the insulin has successfully mopped up most of the glucose circulating in your blood and suddenly you are seriously short of energy, a condition known as rebound hypoglycaemia. You can avoid this state of affairs if you eat carbohydrate every two hours, as I suggest in my eating plan, to keep the blood sugar level even.

Apart from the inconvenience and discomfort of the headache that follows eating excess sucrose, it is potentially dangerous, even if you are not diabetic. As your blood sugar level plummets, you become irritable, impatient, short-tempered. Your concentration goes and so does your ability to make decisions. Your condition deteriorates (viz. the boss after a liquid lunch). Feelings of euphoria and lightheadedness are the prelude to blackout and unconsciousness in extreme cases. In less serious form, the typical response may be to eat another chocolate, gain quick and temporary relief but also start the whole cycle off again.

Therapeutic diets for diabetes are most revealing. Since the diabetic cannot rely on his or her body's own insulin supply to regulate blood sugar, the modern emphasis is towards supplying sugars in slow-release form – as unprocessed carbohydrates, in other words as fresh fruit, vegetables and wholemeal foods. Even if you are not a diabetic, there are good reasons to feed the body's regulating mechanism with a steady influx of sugars from bulky wholefoods, so that insulin need only be used for fine tuning.

That's fine in theory, you may say, but what about my sweet tooth? Carbohydrate craving is the bane of many of us, dieters and non-dieters alike. In the last few years, studies of obese people have suggested a possible basis of the craving and, in doing so, offer us a way to avoid it.

Carbohydrate Cravings, Serotonin and Appetite

It's a common mistake to assume that all obese people are simply greedy and eat anything they can lay their hands on. It's also a mistake to assume that they eat more food than other people at mealtimes. Richard and Judith Wurtman of the Massachusetts Institute of Technology have found that up to two-thirds of all obese people may eat normal-sized meals but then supplement that diet with binges of carbohydrate-rich snacks. A fascinating puzzle that links people's moods with what they eat is beginning to unravel.

Studies show that carbohydrate cravers typically snack in the late afternoon and early evening. If protein-rich food is available as an alternative it is ignored. There must be few of us who don't appreciate the odd biscuit or bun occasionally but, whereas that may satisfy the appetite, carbohydrate cravers continue to eat until they may easily have consumed snacks with the calorific value of a large meal. These snacks are over and above the body's energy needs and, because they invariably consist of refined carbohydrates, i.e. are sugar-rich, they are likely to be converted into fat. Incidentally, these quick and easy snacks were often quick and easy to forget when subjects in the Massachusetts trial were asked to list their daily food intake!

This pattern of excessive eating may already be sounding all too familiar to a great many of you. But, if research from both America and Europe is correct, the kind of food you eat and when you eat it are directly related to your mood.

For most people, eating a snack rich in sugar when they're feeling hungry triggers off the insulin response which leads to rebound hypoglycaemia (albeit mild) with tiredness and sleepiness (see page 151). In sharp contrast, most carbohydrate cravers feel better and refreshed, so they can end up eating more carbohydrates simply for the good feeling it induces.

Many carbohydrate cravers show a marked susceptibility to depression. Not surprisingly, cravers hardly ever eat because of hunger but very often because of fatigue, anxiety or tension. Carbohydrate makes them feel calmer and more clear-headed. Do carbohydrates act as an anti-depressant? Do cravers eat carbohydrates to improve their mood? A bit of brain biochemistry might help to answer some of these questions and to clarify the mystery of appetite.

As we know, the immediate response to a carbohydrate binge is the release of large amounts of insulin into the bloodstream. An indirect consequence of this is that more of that amino-acid, tryptophan, gets into the brain. There it is converted into serotonin, one of the brain's messenger molecules, which makes connections between different nervous networks.

Serotonin appears to act on the 'satiety centre' which is in control of appetite for carbohydrates. In practice, once you have had a couple of biscuits, the sugar from them gets quickly into the bloodstream, insulin is released, more tryptophan gets into the brain and is synthesised into serotonin, and the serotonin floods the control centre, switching off the craving. That's the normal response.

Perhaps with cravers this feedback system doesn't work as quickly to turn off their appetite, or perhaps the switch isn't activated until the level of serotonin is much higher. Or it may simply be that cravers eat to adjust their mood and appetite doesn't come into it. But serotonin is a potent messenger. Drugs that mimic the effect of serotonin but with prolonged action can suppress the snacking behaviour in carbohydrate cravers and facilitate weight loss. Interestingly they can also help in a condition known as seasonal affective disorder where clinical depression is often linked with overeating.

Another important observation is the adverse effect of some other anti-depressant drugs. By blocking the action of serotonin they can induce craving behaviour and so may encourage weight gain. The studies of the Wurtmans and other researchers promise to reveal even more of the secrets underlying the associations between mood and appetite. Many more questions remain to be answered but already we can draw some preliminary conclusions.

My own personal weight-loss diet tries to anticipate carbohydrate craving by scheduling an *unprocessed* starch meal around late afternoon when your blood glucose level may be dropping. This slow-release form of carbohydrate (I suggest some rice or dahl) should help to turn off the craving without resort to sugary snacks (which may exacerbate it). It's important not to eat these carbohydrate-rich snacks with foods that are rich in protein. The more protein that is digested at the same time, the less tryptophan gets through to the brain to make serotonin.

The physiological theory behind this eating plan is sound and logical. It helps you to see why so many diets are bound to fail – they naturally have failure built into them because they make it so hard for the body to control appetite, avoid cravings and binges and eat healthily. On the other hand, this eating plan has a high chance of success because it works with your body and promotes sensible eating.

Eating Plans
for Special
Times in Your
Life

Puberty and Adolescence

A teenager's calorie needs are quite high as most youngsters are still growing and spend a lot of physical and mental energy both at school and in their social life. Of course, how much a teenager eats depends on their age, their size, their sex and their level of activity, but most are eating as much as adults and sometimes more.

If you are concerned about the way your teenager is eating then it is worth while trying to make meals attractive, particularly the all-important breakfast. The easiest way is to change menus frequently. Wholegrain cereals, skimmed milk, fruit yoghurt and low-fat cottage cheese make a nutritious meal but eating exactly the same food every day is boring for everyone, including your teenager. So it is worth providing them with a choice of two cereals, several kinds of fruit, different toppings for pancakes or waffles. You can also make breakfast interesting by offering food that is not usually served at this time such as cheese or peanut butter sandwiches made with wholemeal bread. Cheeseburgers or even nutritious leftovers from dinner can be much more interesting than cereal and eggs.

You may find it easier to get your teenager to eat if you ask them to plan the menus for a week at a time, making a chart and putting it up on the kitchen notice-board.

During adolescence children reach a rate of growth second only to that of infancy. As a result of changes in the composition of their bodies their nutritional needs change. They also differ according to sex. The growth spurt usually begins and ends earlier in girls than in boys so that any dietary recommendations should be used only as guidelines. See table below for recommended protein and energy needs of teenagers according to age, height and weight. Remember, you are the last person to affect your teenagers eating habits. Far and away the greatest influence comes from their peers; consequently family meals assume much less importance than they did when they were younger. Eating becomes a social ritual with their friends and they quite often like to exert greater control over their choice of foods by breaking some of the rules you encouraged at home.

Your adolescent would be unusual if he or she were not concerned about their size, shape and image. Boys very often want to increase their weight. Teenage girls nearly always want to decrease theirs and so many teenage girls are cut-

Recommended Dietary Allowances for Energy and Protein

Sex	Male		Female	
Age	11–14	15–18	11–14	15–18
Weight				
(kg)	44.5	60.0	44.5	54.0
(stones)	7	9½	7	8½
Height				
(cm)	158	172	155	162
(in)	63	69	62	65
Energy				
(calories)	2800	3000	2400	2100
Protein				
(g)	44	54	44	48
(oz)	1.5	1.9	1.5	1.7

ting calories; unfortunately many of them try to reduce their calorie intake by excluding nutritious foods such as bread, cereals and meat, filling up on empty high calorie snacks and soft drinks. More than one in ten girls may be trying to control her weight by some means or other, a few of which are very unhealthy; others, which can lead to anorexia or bulimia, are positively dangerous. If your teenager is overweight and wants to go on a diet make sure that it is a sensible one such as the one given on pages 163–4.

Surveys of teenagers show that eating patterns change so that they stop eating set meals and tend to snack. One of the things that you will have to do, therefore, is to provide a lot of very healthy snacks (see pages 43–4) and salad ingredients (see page 35–7) in the house. Breakfast and lunch are the meals most often skipped – especially by girls on diets; but patterns may also become irregular because of school activities, social demands and part-time jobs. Because of this a teenager may take in well over what she or he needs in nutrients one day and well under the next. Try to keep a sense of balance and remember that it is not necessary to meet all food requirements every day as long as the teenager has an adequate intake over a period of about a week.

There is incontrovertible evidence that adolescents can get all the nutrients they need from healthy snacks. Some of the junk foods that adults usually malign are not as lacking in nutrition as you may think. None the less they should still be eaten only occasionally rather than forming the main part of the diet. Armed with the tables on pages 165–7, which shows you the amount of food from each food group an adolescent needs, you can now apply the principles of my eating plan to your teenagers' needs. Good luck!

A Balanced Low-Calorie Diet for Adolescents

Breakfast	Calories
1 serving fruit or juice	40
175 g (6 oz) wholegrain ready-to-eat cereal	75
225 ml (8 fl oz) skimmed milk	120
1 slice wholegrain bread	60
1 teaspoon margarine or butter	45
Total	340

Lunch	Calories
50 g (2 oz) lean meat, cheese or fish	175
2 slices wholewheat bread	120
1 teaspoon margarine or butter	45
1 serving vegetable or fruit	40
225 ml (8 fl oz) skimmed milk	120
Total	500

Dinner	Calories
75 g (3 oz) lean meat, fish, poultry or other protein food	250
1 serving vegetable	40
1 salad	40
1 small potato or 125 g (4 oz) rice or noodles or 1 slice wholewheat bread	80
1 teaspoon margarine or butter	45
1 serving fruit	40
225 ml (8 fl oz) skimmed milk	120
Total	615
Meals total	1455

Snacks (Optional)	Calories
1 serving fruit	40
125 g (4 oz) ice-cream or 1 small cup-cake with icing or 3 small biscuits	125
Total	165
Day's total	1620

Daily Food Guide

Cereals and Grains

Wholegrain breads and cereals, brown rice, wholewheat pasta.

	Number of Servings	1-serving Equivalent
3–5 years	4 or more	½–1 slice bread 1 tablespoon cereal × years of age
6–10 years	4 or more	1 slice bread 125–225 g (4–8 oz) cereal
11–18 years	4 or more	1 slice bread 125–225 g (4–8 oz) cereal

Fruits and Vegetables

All fruits and vegetables. Be sure to include some dark-green or yellow vegetables for vitamin A and some citrus fruits or other source of vitamin C.

	Number of Servings	1-serving Equivalent
3–5 years	4 or more	1 small fruit or vegetable 50–125 g (2–4 oz)
6–10 years	4 or more	1 medium fruit or vegetable 125–150 g (4–5 oz)
11–18 years	4 or more	1 medium fruit or vegetable 125–225 g (4–8 oz)

Meat, Fish and Eggs

Lean meats, fish, poultry, eggs, dried peas and beans. One egg or 125 g (4 oz) peas/beans or 2 tablespoons peanut butter is equal to 25 g (1 oz) of meat.

	Number of Servings	1-serving Equivalent
3–5 years	2 or more	25–75 g (1–3 oz) meat
6–10 years	2 or more	50–125 g (2–4 oz) meat
11–18 years	2 or more	75–125 g (3–4 oz) meat, fish or poultry

Milk and Dairy Products

Semi-skimmed and skimmed milk, natural yoghurt, ice-cream, cheese and other dairy products.

	Number of Servings	1-serving Equivalent
3–5 years	2–3	125–225 ml (4–8 fl oz) milk
6–10 years	under 9: 2–3 over 9: 3 or more	225 ml (8 fl oz) milk
11–18 years	3 or more	225 ml (8 fl oz) milk

A Healthy Diet for Pregnant Women and Nursing Mothers

The seven-day diet given at the front of the book is so well balanced that it is perfectly safe for pregnant women and nursing mothers to embark upon. In fact it is probably better than the average diet that most women usually eat. It follows, therefore, that on this healthy, well-balanced diet you will only have to make minor adjustments to accommodate any increased nutritional needs when you are pregnant. Remember it is essential that you do not smoke during pregnancy and most doctors recommend that you do not drink alcohol.

A basic rule is that you should never try to lose weight when you are pregnant and while it is normal to eat slightly more than usual during pregnancy it is not an excuse for over-eating – you should never 'eat for two'. In general your energy requirements increase by about 15 per cent which means that you do need more calories, but only 150 more calories a day in the first three months, 300 a day in the second trimester, and 400 to 450 in the last trimester.

Most women who are pregnant experience an increase in appetite. However, your digestive system is slowing down and during the last trimester your stomach takes longer to empty because the baby is pushing against it. It is important for your comfort as well as your digestion therefore not to overload the stomach, so my initial eating plan of five to six small meals a day is much better suited to a pregnant woman than eating a smaller number of larger meals.

For the healthy development of your baby your daily diet needs to contain adequate protein, calcium, phosphorus, iodine, iron and vitamins A, B, C and D. Here is a table which shows you which foods contain these nutrients:

* Milk and dairy products: a high percentage of the protein, most of the calcium and phosphorus, and all of the vitamin D.
* Meat, fish and poultry: a lot of protein, B vitamins and some iron.
* Vegetables, potatoes and citrus fruits: some protein and large quantities of vitamin C; vegetables are also an excellent source of vitamin A.
* Grains and cereals: iron and B vitamins, and smaller amounts of protein, calcium and phosphorus.

While you are pregnant your baby requires a lot of liquid because the blood volume expands in order to nourish the baby so it is a good idea to drink about two pints of skimmed milk a day and about three pints of other liquid. When you are breast-feeding you will need another four pints. Avoid fizzy drinks and cut back on tea and coffee – they all contain caffeine which may not be good for the unborn baby; and do not forget that when you drink tea with a meal the tannic acid in it can prevent your digestion from absorbing iron from the food.

Fresh, unprocessed foods have the highest nutritional value. It may also be harmful to eat a lot of foods that contain chemical preservatives, colourings and flavourings. Therefore, eat as much raw food as you possibly can and buy lots of fresh fruit and vegetables. Do not eat any food that is stale or has mould on it. Cutting off the mould does not always remove the toxins which may have penetrated deeper into the food and which are not destroyed by cooking.

Avoid canned, frozen and packaged convenience foods, processed meats such as sausage and commercial pâtés, products made with refined flour, bottled sauces and pickles and high calorie snacks such as crisps, biscuits and sweets. Avoid raw eggs and only eat eggs which are cooked sufficiently for the white to be quite firm.

If you follow all these rules you will avoid ingesting salmonella, listeria and campylobacter. You will also be eating a healthy diet for both you and your baby.

Food for the Over-fifties

It is very important that you should continue to eat a varied and well-balanced diet as you get older. As a general rule, however, you will be less active than you were when you were younger so you burn up fewer calories and therefore need less food. As you age, the digestive system slows down so you will be much more comfortable if you eat smaller meals and more snacks very much along the lines of the diet given at the beginning of the book.

Your diet should concentrate on unprocessed fresh carbohydrates in the form of fresh fruit and vegetables, potatoes, wholegrain breads and cereals. Eat lots of calcium-rich foods such as those shown in the table on page 173.

Food Providing 200 mg Calcium

Cheese, hard	25 g	1 oz
Sardines	50 g	2 oz
Yoghurt, low-fat	125 g	4 oz
Skimmed milk	175 ml	6 fl oz
Bread, white	225 g	8 oz
Peanuts	350 g	12 oz
Cabbage, cooked	450 g	16 oz

As you get older, warm foods and beverages become easier to digest than cold ones. You also need plenty of liquids every day. So soups and stews provide tasty ways to fulfil most of your nutritional requirements.

With increasing age we tend to become absent-minded and it is easy to neglect the diet. If you find this is your problem you must devise ways to overcome it. So, for example, impose set mealtimes on yourself and plan all your meals and snacks a day at a time. Do it first thing in the morning after breakfast and put the menus on the kitchen notice-board. Another way to prompt yourself about eating is to have at least one snack a day with a friend, a neighbour or a member of the family, or possibly with your favourite television programme or while you listen to the radio. Make a firm resolve to do so.

Even if you have never eaten a healthy diet before, it is never too late to start. Set yourself realistic goals and adapt to changes in your diet very gradually, only making one change (such as swopping from whole milk to skimmed milk) per week. If you think it is going to be difficult remember that you learned your old food preferences so you can unlearn them and learn new ones. You do not have to give up any food entirely (see the 80/20 rule on page 92) but be sure to tell your family and friends the changes that you are making to your diet and ask them to support you.

After retirement we usually have less disposable income and so it is very important that we get value for money while we are buying food. The following table may help you to make some prudent decisions – both for your purse and for your health!

Value For Money

	More Nutrition for Your Money	Less Nutrition for Your Money
Meat	Poultry: chicken, turkey Game: pheasant, pigeon, partridge, rabbit, venison Liver and other offal Home-made burgers and meat products from lean minced steak or other meat Low-fat sausages	Pork, beef, lamb Meat pies and pasties Luncheon meat Manufactured burgers, meat pâtés, spreads and speciality sausages Standard sausages and sausage-meat

	More Nutrition for Your Money	**Less Nutrition for Your Money**
Fish	Plain frozen fish (no additives) Home-made fish fingers and fish cakes Wet fish, canned tuna, sardines and mackerel	Fish frozen with poly-phosphates or in sauces Manufactured fish fingers and other fish in batter Canned fish in sauces and canned shellfish
Bread and Cereals	Breads: wholemeal, wheatgerm, granary, mixed-grain, sprouted-seed, pumpernickel and rye Sugar-free breakfast cereals Porridge	White bread and rolls Croissants and other sweet-ened breads Breakfast cereals con-taining sugar, salt and food colouring Instant hot cereals

	More Nutrition for Your Money	**Less Nutrition for Your Money**
Fats	Soft vegetable margarines high in poly-unsaturates, Unsalted butter Polyunsaturated vegetable oils e.g. sunflower, safflower, corn Home-made salad dressings e.g. French dressing, vinaigrette	Hard and soft margarines low in poly-unsaturates, dairy spreads, low-fat spreads Salted butter Dripping, lard, suet, blended unspecified cooking oils Bottled or other ready-made salad dressings

	More Nutrition for Your Money	**Less Nutrition for Your Money**
Vegetables	Fresh fruit and vegetables in season Fruit canned in its own juice Vegetables canned without added salt or sugar Plain frozen vegetables Fresh potatoes	Bruised and overripe fruit and vegetables Fruit canned in syrup Vegetables canned with salt and/or sugar Frozen vegetables in sauces Frozen chips, potato products in batter
Drinks	Milk – see above Fruit juices, fresh and reconstituted Naturally carbonated fruit juices and mineral water with added juice	Milk – see above Fruit-flavoured drinks and squash Fizzy drinks with added sugar or artificial sweeteners, colours and flavours

	More Nutrition for Your Money	**Less Nutrition for Your Money**
Dairy Produce	Mature and farmhouses cheeses	Mild cheeses, processed cheeses and cheese slices
	Edam, Gouda and reduced-fat hard cheeses	Blue cheeses and some flavoured cheeses
	Unsweetened and natural yoghurt, low-fat yoghurt	Full-fat yoghurt Fruit-flavoured yoghurt
	Real fruit yoghurt	Full-fat milk and milk with extra fat
	Skimmed and semi-skimmed milk	Dried milk with added fats
	Dried skimmed milk	

GOOD HOUSEKEEPING

EATING FOR A HEALTHY
Skin

ALIX KIRSTA

GOOD HOUSEKEEPING
— the recipe for healthy living

Do sweets really cause spots?
Is eczema food-related?
Does vitamin E prevent ageing?

Working on the principle that we are what we eat,
GOOD HOUSEKEEPING EATING FOR A HEALTHY
SKIN answers all these questions and more while
showing how healthy eating can make a real
difference to the way we look.

With a wide range of delicious recipes high in the
nutrients essential for a good-looking skin, GOOD
HOUSEKEEPING EATING FOR A HEALTHY SKIN
covers everything from Breakfast and Brunch to
Seasonal Salads, Puddings and Desserts.
But this is more than just a recipe book. It also
provides invaluable information on all aspects of skin
care, from preventing spots to avoiding allergies, and
gives sound advice on how best to withstand such perils
of everyday life as stress and exposure to sun
and pollution. Eat for a healthy skin and eat
for a healthy life.

More Cookery from Headline:

GOOD HOUSEKEEPING

EATING FOR A HEALTHY

Heart

WITH THE CORONARY PREVENTION GROUP

GOOD HOUSEKEEPING
— the recipe for healthy living

**Low in fat, sugar and salt, high in fibre —
and absolutely delicious!**

From breakfasts and brunches to dinner parties,
picnics and barbecues — the 250 recipes in this
mouthwatering collection show you how to cook
healthily for every occasion. And with low-fat
variations on such family favourites as moussaka
and Cornish pasties — plus delicious new dishes like
lamb fillet with leek sauce and chilled vanilla soufflé
— it contains all you need to entice even the most
unhealthy of palates to abandon the (bad)
habits of a lifetime.

Each recipe is accompanied by an analysis of its
nutritional value; the introduction provides reams of
invaluable information on the prevention of
coronary heart disease based on years of medical
research. Eat the dishes and follow the guidelines —
and you and your family can reduce the risk of
heart disease and look forward to a
longer and healthier life.

'A very practical book' *Woman's Realm*

'Gives all the recipes, nutritional information and
advice that one would practically need' *Taste*

NON-FICTION/COOKERY   0 7472 3278 4   £3.99

A selection of bestsellers from Headline

FICTION		
BLOOD STOCK	John Francome & James MacGregor	£3.99 □
THE OLD SILENT	Martha Grimes	£4.50 □
ALL THAT GLITTERS	Katherine Stone	£4.50 □
A FAMILY MATTER	Nigel Rees	£4.50 □
EGYPT GREEN	Christopher Hyde	£4.50 □

NON-FICTION		
MY MOUNTBATTEN YEARS	William Evans	£4.50 □
WICKED LADY Salvador Dali's Muse	Tim McGirk	£4.99 □
THE FOOD OF SPAIN AND PORTUGAL	Elisabeth Lambert Ortiz	£5.99 □

SCIENCE FICTION AND FANTASY		
REVENGE OF THE FLUFFY BUNNIES Cineverse Cycle Book 3	Craig Shaw Gardner	£3.50 □
BROTHERS IN ARMS	Lois McMaster Bujold	£4.50 □
THE SEA SWORD	Adrienne Martine-Barnes	£3.50 □
NO HAVEN FOR THE GUILTY	Simon Green	£3.50 □
GREENBRIAR QUEEN	Sheila Gilluly	£4.50 □

All Headline books are available at your local bookshop or newsagent, or can be ordered direct from the publisher. Just tick the titles you want and fill in the form below. Prices and availability subject to change without notice.

Headline Book Publishing PLC, Cash Sales Department, PO Box 11, Falmouth, Cornwall, TR10 9EN, England.

Please enclose a cheque or postal order to the value of the cover price and allow the following for postage and packing:
UK: 80p for the first book and 20p for each additional book ordered up to a maximum charge of £2.00
BFPO: 80p for the first book and 20p for each additional book
OVERSEAS & EIRE: £1.50 for the first book, £1.00 for the second book and 30p for each subsequent book.

Name ....

Address ....

....

....